SHIT HAPPENS

THE MICROBIOME STORY

THOMAS J BORODY

ISBN: 978-0-6457859-4-4 (hardback)
ISBN: 978-0-6457859-5-1 (paperback)
ISBN: 978-0-6457859-3-7 (e-book)

First edition 2025
Published by Bouley Bay Books, Sydney & Jersey
www.bouleybaybooks.com
Typeset and printed in Australia by Image DTO
imagedto@gmail.com
Cover design by Trish Le Moignan
Copyright © Professor Thomas J Borody, Australia (2025)

This book is dedicated to all the medical researchers and their patients who have had the courage and foresight to venture where no-one had dared to go before, risking their lives, health and wellbeing to find new treatments or cures for all the many ailments that flesh is heir to.

No man is an island and few books are the work of any one person. Professor Thomas Borody acknowledges with gratitude the valuable assistance he has received from Dr Siba Dolai and Dr Will Davies.

CONTENTS

Foreword 6

Introduction 9

1 Discovering the microbiome 21

2 Seeing and studying the microbiome 29

3 What is the microbiome? 33

4 The microbiome under attack 39

5 The microbiome's defence 45

6 The microbiome recovers 47

7 Other microbiome communities in nature 53

8 The current view of the microbiome 57

9 How gut bacteria evolved with the human body 61

10 A microbiome theory of disease 65

11 The first silver bullet: Josie and FMT 69

12 Recognising *Clostridium difficile* infection 73

13 Ensuring safety of FMT for wider *C. difficile* treatment 77

14 The case against microbes 81

15 Paving the way forward 85

16 Differences between *Helicobacter* and *C. difficile* 91

17 Crossing the great divide 97

18 MS reversed in mice and men 101

19 FMT's effects on Parkinson's and Alzheimer's 107

20 The challenge of autism 113

21 Advancing medical knowledge - risky but rewarding 119

22 Treatments old and new 123

23 Dealing with dysbiosis 129

24 The microbiome and YOU 137

References 141

Acknowledgements 153

FOREWORD

Shit! You can't get away from it. This is a shit book, from start to finish. It's all about shit – shit, we're full of it. We all shit, we talk shit, behave shit, sometimes we even look shit.

Shit is one of the most overused, underrated and versatile words in the English language. It made up over 25% of the 38 words in the previous paragraph, appearing variously as noun, verb, adjective, adverb, conjunction and (initially) as an exclamation/expletive.

If this very common Anglo-Saxon monosyllabic offends or upsets you, just mentally replace it with faeces, crap, excrement, poo, poop, bowel movement, number twos, stools, defecation, discharge, dung, doodoos or whichever euphemism you prefer. But don't be deceived: compared with the succinct original, they're all shit.

We all do it. Even birds and bees do it. Every living thing that takes in sustenance excretes waste matter. We humans are unique in loathing this most natural substance. All of our five senses are highly trained to repel it. We hate the sight of it, the smell, sound, texture – our stomachs would turn over at the thought of tasting it.

We all produce about the same amount of it, almost every day of our lives, and then we go to enormous lengths to transport it miles away from us, preferably without smelling, touching or looking at it.

This book describes the recent, extraordinary discovery that this apparently lifeless waste matter can inform us, if we will only listen, whether we are sick or well – and what, specifically, is wrong with us.

Our faeces teem with life. They are stuffed with millions and millions of different microbes, the vast majority of which are yet to be identified.

The condition of the microbiome of our gut, which produces this thriving waste matter, determines whether we suffer several debilitating, maybe fatal conditions. Irregularities in our microbiota can certainly cause or intensify diarrhea, constipation, colitis, coeliac disease, peptic and duodenal ulcers, irritable bowel syndrome, inflammatory bowel disease, colon cancer, periodontal disease, atherosclerosis, endocarditis and other gastric complaints, and may be influential in obesity, anxiety and depression – but there are strong indications that they may also be responsible for (or at least exacerbate) a wide variety of currently 'incurable' illnesses, such as Type 2 Diabetes, Multiple Sclerosis, Parkinson's, Alzheimer's and Crohn's Disease and Autism. The good news is that, if we get our shit together, we can reverse or cure many of these conditions and live healthier, happier lives.

The discoveries of the first antibiotic, penicillin, and the horde of other antibiotics that followed were undoubtedly a great boon and blessing for mankind – but these antibiotics have also presented our microbiota with unprecedented challenges, which medical practitioners and researchers are only just beginning to understand.

The human biome (the universe of living beings inside every one of us) is still something of a mystery, even to experts who are studying it. It developed over millions of years, as a symbiotic relationship between the human hosts and the multitude of microbial tenants. They enabled us to digest and draw benefits from all manner of foodstuffs which helped us to be stronger, live longer, stretch, move, act and think more effectively. Our gut is home to a vastly greater variety of living creatures than any other natural habitat on earth.

For centuries, we have searched for the sources of illnesses outside of ourselves: now, we are beginning to understand that many diseases originate in the microbial soup sloshing about in our own bodies. We are learning to consume more and more foods with prebiotic or probiotic qualities. Using antibiotics to suppress undesirable conditions may inadvertently weaken our defences against other, potentially more serious ailments. It's common sense to try and make them stronger.

Brilliant medical researchers and practitioners like Professor Thomas Borody are pioneering radical, new techniques to replace our own, sick shit with healthy shit that will extend our lives and make them worth living. This book tells the stories behind these life-changing discoveries and tries to forecast how their application may change the course of medical practice in the future beyond all recognition.

Mick Le Moignan

INTRODUCTION

Starting my Microbiome Journey

For those readers who do not know me, please allow me to introduce myself. Alternatively, if you are keen to get to the 'nitty gritty' of this book, feel free to skip to Chapter One, *The discovery of the microbiome*.

When I came to medicine as a young undergraduate at the University of NSW in 1969, the word 'microbiome' did not exist. While there is some conjecture as to the first use of the word, it is generally accepted that Dr. John M. Whipps first coined it in 1988. At that time, I was already exploring the microbiome in detail with faecal microbiota transplants - FMT.

My journey in medicine has always involved trying to understand microbiota in humans. It has been a long road, and I invite you to join me in reflecting on this journey. Much has happened, much research has been undertaken, much has been learned and enormous benefits to mankind have ensued. This includes the now completed Human Microbiome Project, a United States National Institute of Health project started in 2007 to improve our understanding of the microbiome and its role in human health and disease prevention. However, this is just a small part of the work carried out over the past fifty years in this field of medicine, including the research and treatments undertaken by myself and my colleagues at the Centre for Digestive Diseases in Sydney.

Today, I and my team at the Centre are continuing to explore the mysterious world of the microbiome. We are also keen to explain to people what the microbiome is and how we can help you to improve your health.

In this little book, there are answers to your stomach problems and a range of medical questions that stem from gut issues, but first, let me explain how I came to study this subject. It has occupied and preoccupied me for most of my life and I still find it fascinating and absorbing…

My story begins after my family were fortunate to get out of Communist Poland and find a new life in Australia in early 1960. After high school, I was privileged to get a scholarship to study Medicine at the University of NSW in Kensington, Sydney in 1969. Here, I found I enjoyed pathology. I was introduced to histological sections, the study of human tissue and organs through sectioning, staining and then examining samples on a glass slide under a microscope. Here for the first time was the human microbiome laid out for me to explore. Little did I know at the time that this intriguing biological conundrum would provide the impetus for my life's work.

While still at UNSW, I travelled to Prince Henry Hospital to work with my tutor, Dr Cummings, who demonstrated how to open the skull and carefully reveal the brain. For me, this was an emotional and testing time, confronted as I was with the mortality of man, on the one hand, while on the other, the wonder of the advanced human machine, intricate, efficient and highly evolved, a bag of smelly parts – the human microbiome laid bare.

After three years of Medicine, I completed my BSc (Med) in pathology in 1972, as this further study would provide me with an extra qualification and prepare me for the research process ahead. Fortunately, I could afford to do it, because I was one year younger than my fellow students and had money coming in from driving cabs and selling cars. However, I had little time for recreation and now found myself virtually living at the university, sleeping in a storeroom on a pile of old curtains on the floor.

After completing the BSc (Med) my medical studies became a lot easier. I read avidly, and it was all distinctions and high distinctions after that. Graduating with my MB BS, (Bachelor of Medicine and Bachelor of Surgery) in 1974, I worked as a doctor at the Army's 2nd Military District Hospital at Ingleburn in southwestern Sydney, treating military personnel, including casualties from the Vietnam War.

Following graduation, I became a medical intern and was given the choice of taking a medical as opposed to a surgical path. I chose the medical path, where I would rotate through surgery, respiratory, cardiology, intensive care, ER and other areas. I did at times undertake surgical procedures, but I found I was not interested in a purely surgical future. Perhaps it was the early interest and encouragement I had received in pathology that set the path for my later specialist research work in gastroenterology and the human microbiome.

Post-graduation, I worked for a term as a medical intern at the Royal Hospital for Women in Paddington, under senior people like Dr Alex Szirt, along with doctors Cliff Rosendahl and Rod Peek, who wrote *The Handbook of Obstetrics and Gynecology,* edited by Professor Barry Wren, first published in 1975. In February of that year, I began my residency at St Vincent's Hospital in Darlinghurst, in inner Sydney. It was here that I met an important mentor, Dr James Hayes, who introduced me to renal medicine and dialysis. Jim Hayes was such a gentleman and gave me one of my most memorable learning experiences. He would never get angry and stayed calm, even when his students failed to understand.

Another specialist at St Vincent's who had a profound effect on my later career was Dr Dudley O'Sullivan, a superb neurologist who studied disorders in the nervous system and treated a range of conditions that affect the brain, spinal cord and nerves. He was the best neurologist I have ever come across. He taught me diagnosis in neurology and how it is rarely achieved by doing a blood test. Much more effective is a physical examination, starting with the cranial nerves, to identify problems and to test tone, power, coordination, reflexes, walking and handshake relaxation.

The pressure on young interns was and still is enormous. After my cardiology and intensive care rotations, I was frequently scheduled to be part of the hospital's cardiac arrest resuscitation team, where I did many resuscitations, I guess in the hundreds. The pressure of daily work plus being on-call with the resuscitation team meant that I rarely had an uninterrupted sleep. I always had to be ready. Sometimes I'd wake up in the middle of the night, call the switchboard and say

'Where's the cardiac arrest? I think I slept through it!' and they'd say, 'there was no cardiac arrest, you must have dreamt it.' I'd be so relieved. It was an awful feeling, thinking you might have let somebody down. But there were some lighter moments. I remember when we resuscitated an Italian man and someone called out 'Mr. Sergi, this is Saint Peter, you are in heaven!' We were naughty - we were a lot younger then.

In my second year of residency at St Vincent's, I needed to decide my future area of specialist medicine. I was working under two inspirational gastroenterologists, Dr David Byrnes and Dr Bill Hennessy. Dr Byrnes had an interest in research at the Garvan Institute, especially in gastrointestinal hormones, and he found me a place to work in his lab. It was working with these two men that helped me to make up my mind. I was wondering whether to do cardiology, endocrinology or respiratory medicine. I settled on gastroenterology. I realised gastroenterological procedures did not need a hospital surgical ward and so could be done at separate, private clinics across the city. At that time, none were operating, so Bill Hennessy, David Byrnes and I set up our own private clinic in Victoria Street, Darlinghurst, near the famous Bar Coluzzi.

I was now for the first time in an ambitious, groundbreaking, professional medical practice with celebrated medical colleagues, undertaking operations outside the traditional hospital system. I put together an endoscopy room at the back, which could be entered through a garage door from the street behind, and a recovery room where we were sedating people and endoscoping them. This gave me an extraordinary and focused start to what would become a very special medical career. But there was one more experience, one more place to go and from it came some unique and incisive answers to medical conundrums that would come up in my pioneering work ahead.

By the end of 1977, I had completed my three years as a medical intern resident and registrar, had married and had a baby daughter, Julie. I was looking for another challenge. After speaking with my gastroenterological mentor, Bill Hennessy, I became interested in tropical medicine. Bill was an expert in this area and told stories of his time in New Guinea and the medical frontiers there. Inspired by this conversation, my mind turned to where my wife Sue and I might emulate Bill's experience, within the Seventh Day Adventist medical missionary service. I found the church had a medical facility in the Pacific, and their mission and hospital on Malaita in the Solomon Islands became our home for the next year.

The first excitement of our Solomons adventure happened, 3000 feet in the air, when the aircraft's engine stopped. We were in a small aeroplane just big enough for the four of us: myself, my wife Sue, our tiny baby Julie in a basket next to me and the pilot. The engine sound died, to be replaced only by the rolling swoosh of the air off the wings – or was it the palm trees below? Our stomachs dropped and the jungle-clad island stretched before us, but as the plane lost altitude, we glided closer and closer to the open sea. The aircraft had floats, so I crossed my fingers and began to hope we could land in the water instead. As I ran through these scenarios and nervously rocked Julie beside me, the pilot flicked a switch, and the engine roared back to life. Turning around, he said casually, 'Oh, we always do this. Switching the wing gas tank from right to left before we land.' I didn't say anything. When we finally landed, my heart was still in my throat.

Our new home was at the Atoifi Hospital on Malaita, one of the Solomon Islands in the South Pacific Ocean, some 3,000 kilometres or 1,600 nautical miles northeast of Sydney. Malaita is the second largest of the Solomon Islands after Guadalcanal, but the most populated. It is tropical with a mountainous spine, about 100 kilometres long and just 37 kilometres wide. Being right on the Equator, it is hot and extremely wet, with a fickle weather pattern, heavy rain and high humidity. There are also destructive cyclones and, being part of the Pacific 'ring of fire', the Solomons are also subject to frequent earthquakes. For my wife and myself and our tiny daughter, it was different from Australia and very different again from blizzardy Poland.

We were in Malaita to fill staff shortages after a major incident. A few years before our arrival, the hospital's opening had been delayed by the death of a nurse and missionary worker, Graham Dunn, who had travelled to Malaita with his wife to provide medical support to the people. Before his death, it was reported in the papers that the church had a large holding of land, which had been purchased in 1904 for just forty pounds, but was later revealed to be worth two thousand pounds. The traditional owners, the Kwaio tribe, claimed they were owed the difference for their land, but were refused this remuneration by the church. Not long after, Graham Dunn was speared to death in what was understood at the time to be an act of revenge or 'payback'. It was largely condemned by many Kwaio leaders, but while the hospital did open, it held on by a thread, struggling with the shortage of staff and the necessary medical supplies.

Connected to the hospital was our purpose-built house, made of hollow brick, reinforced with steel rods and cement and topped with a corrugated iron roof. This kind of building was vital because of the earthquakes which happened once a week or so. We knew they were coming because the echoing calls of the tropical birds stopped, and the island became eerily quiet – the calm before the storm. Then the dogs started barking, always followed by the sound of tinkling plates and the banging of our shelves against the walls. It felt like the whole house was rumbling, but we learned to wait for it to pass and pretty soon we got used to the quakes.

Fortunately, the house had ceiling fans. There was no air conditioning at the time and the house, like the hospital, needed serious work and maintenance. It rained torrentially twice a day on the island, but the rain could not cut through the 35-degree heat. I generally woke up every morning sweating as though I was in a sauna. After only a month there, I lost about twelve kilos in bodyweight from the sweltering heat and constant perspiration. I had to keep reminding myself that it was the heat and not the hookworm, which was endemic on the island at the time.

The rest of the house was littered with cases of tinned food and journal articles from home that we had crammed into our suitcases, unsure of what to expect from Malaita. Though the island was home to nearly 80,000 people at the time, there was not a single shop, so we relied on locally caught fish. To help us with baby Julie, we had two 'cookie girls', Janeti and Nedula, who used to carry Julie around on their hips. Julie wore a hibiscus in her hair, the flower so large that it covered one side of her head. She was fascinated by blood, perhaps an early consequence of having two doctors as parents. Often, Janeti or Nedua would bring her to the operating theatre during the day, so she could see her parents at work – and of course, to relish the blood.

Our work began as soon as we arrived at the Atoifi hospital. Everything was new – it was a real challenge. We were in uncharted waters, without the usual hospital staff. We had to shoot our own x-rays, develop them in a dark room and then wait for them to dry so they were readable. My only other experience of this was developing photographs with my parents thirty years earlier. I never thought I would need to apply this knowledge in my medical career. All our x-ray machines were broken in one way or another and x-raying children with serious illnesses was the trickiest. I tried hard to make them understand what I wanted. In the end, we would wait for a screaming child to inhale before they started wailing again, and quickly shoot the x-ray. It was not always easy, but it worked most of the time. Working like this, I was also getting a crash course in the local dialect, Pidgin English, and the local language, Kwaio, although there were said to be over a hundred languages spoken in Malaita.

It seemed everyone on the island was sick. Even moving between a few beds, we would encounter a wide array of diseases. They all had hookworm and malaria, and many patients had tuberculosis. These were diseases that had largely been eradicated in Australia and if found, would quickly be referred to an infectious disease specialist. That wasn't an option here. Instead, we had to learn to recognise all the symptoms and work with what equipment we had to test and treat the patients. There was a small pathology lab, but we did not have to use the lab to diagnose malaria, as we knew it from their clinical description and, if it was worsening, simply from the tell-tale signs of rigors and a 43° fever.

We had a small teaching microscope to assist us with some diagnoses, but there were other challenges. There was no disposable equipment, and supplies were few and far between, so everything had to be sterilised and re-used. From the time we arrived, the clinic had about a hundred patients lined up, waiting, every day. One sign outside on the wall said it was 10 cents to see the doctor, but another below it said 'big sick anytime' – our version of an emergency room.

Many visitors to the clinic were in urgent need of dental work to alleviate severe pain, so I was shown basic procedures by a visiting dentist, Dr Doug Easthope. Doug visited for a week and showed Sue and me how to drill and fill teeth and inject xylocaine. Some of the people who came to the clinic were from the highland areas and arrived completely naked, their teeth pitch black. We had a dentist's chair, but the drill had no water running through it. Nothing that was donated to the hospital was working, and without water, the drill would cause the teeth to burn and the gums to boil, so I had to improvise. With a lumbar puncture needle glued alongside the end of the drill and a line running to an intravenous bag beside the chair, I had a makeshift dentist's drill, cooled by running water. The World Health Organisation provided IV bags by the crate, so at least we had a good supply of them.

We had no telephones and could only communicate sporadically via radio. So, at night I would write letters on an old typewriter to request supplies from Australia. My letters were pleading, 'please send, please donate, please give anything you can.' We needed everything from new toilets to new ceilings. You could hear the rats running across the pipes in the ceilings of the wards and the pharmacy was full of geckos. I would write to the church, to anyone I could for donations. The mail came by seaplane every two to six weeks and this was one of the few ways we could get messages out of the island. I sent many of these letters to the church and a lot of donations came through that way. I also wrote frequently to Sir Reginald Ansett, who was very supportive. He would arrange no-cost flights for the children who needed special operations. Some of the telegrams I sent to Sir Reginald would come back with only a short reply: 'Yes… oxygen and wheelchair waiting.'

The year passed swiftly amidst days of relentless patient demands and an ongoing struggle for supplies. As our time in Malaita neared its conclusion, I resumed planning for my return to Australia, and prepared job applications for my anticipated homecoming to Sydney. With each passing day, it became increasingly apparent that the myriad patient experiences and the broad exposure to various illnesses, ranging from TB to leprosy, had taught me to navigate situations that extended way beyond my primary medical expertise. I performed procedures as though I were a surgeon and learned to administer tooth fillings, despite not being a dentist. From patients experiencing jaw pain to those grappling with TB, Addison's, hookworms, Trichuris infections in the gut and even bowel obstructions, I gained invaluable insights. These experiences equipped me with a profound understanding of a fundamental principle of medicine – the importance of looking for infections wherever inflammation presents itself.

Looking back, my experience in the Solomon Islands was intense, unfamiliar and at times frightening. I was treating diseases I had never seen in Australia, for example, tetanus, and making do with the bare minimum of supplies. That was always the struggle - to do more with a dwindling stock of supplies, especially medications, with no idea when more might come. But my time at Atoifi taught me much: it was here that I really learned medicine. There was no one to ask for help, since there were no telephones. We were constantly overwhelmed, feeling somewhat helpless. Each week brought new challenges and losses - one week, we lost thirty very young children who lived in the mountains, to a widespread bout of diarrhea and extremely severe dehydration. One patient I saw was so dehydrated with sunken eyes, that if you pushed a little on his eye, your finger went into the skull, back towards the brain.

Every day we were treating multiple diseases mixed with something different, a disease with different causes or complications. It was only retrospectively that I realised how important my time in Malaita was in learning how to treat intracellular infections and how much knowledge I gained from treating malaria, TB and leprosy, diseases uncommon in Australia. These were intracellular infections. That is, they resided within human cells and required multiple, concurrent antibiotics that could work within cells.

The diseases I observed on Malaita were incurable with single antibiotic therapies, as the bacteria would simply persist in the patient or develop antimicrobial resistance. Medicine at this point was only based on the concept of extracellular infections, which involved bacteria living in the spaces between or outside of our cells. While extracellular infections could often be addressed with a single antibiotic, as with urinary infections, the notion that bacteria could reside within human cells was entirely revolutionary. But, most important of all, this experience gave me a robust and deep understanding of what would distil in my brain and in my practice treating the human microbiome. The realisation that concealed pathogens could induce persistent chronic inflammation, potentially leading to cancer, would become a recurring theme that was encountered by numerous researchers. These innovative ideas and concepts would lead to several Nobel Prizes in the years ahead.

Back in Australia, my St Vincent's Hospital mentor, Dr David Byrnes, had become increasingly interested in intestinal health and 'gut hormones' and spoke to Dr Lazarus, one of the founders of the Garvan Institute within St. Vincent's Hospital, suggesting that I be invited to do a doctorate of Medicine there. I worked in Dr Byrnes' lab at the Garvan in gut hormones and motility, resulting in a doctorate of Medicine by thesis. This was the first of my three doctorates, working initially on gastrointestinal hormones and motility. After two years at the Garvan, I realised I needed overseas experience and, again with the help of Dr David Byrnes, was able to secure an introduction to an Australian gastroenterologist working at the famous Mayo Clinic in Rochester, Minnesota, Professor Sid Phillips. To fund this trip, I was fortunate to be awarded a Neil Hamilton-Fairley Fellowship and so Sue, four-year-old Julie and I set off for Rochester, arriving there in February 1981.

The Mayo Clinic was originally founded by Dr William Mayo, a surgeon in the Union Army during the Civil War. To survive, he operated a ferry service, became a farmer, worked as a GP and, in the process, established a small medical research clinic. This became the Mayo Foundation in the early 1920s. It was in this amazing and enduring institution that I and my family found ourselves living and working. By this time, the Mayo Clinic was massive, employing a large percentage of the town's population (34,180 employees in 2016) and was the core of the town's economy. Yet, while the summers were warm, Rochester was the second windiest city in the country, with freezing winters down to -40° Celsius and heavy snow, an enormous change for us from Sydney.

Along with Professor Sid Phillips, I initially worked on human motility because it had been the subject of my doctorate, but I found the Mayo was far behind in many aspects of medicine. Then I moved into gallstone dissolution with a friend of mine, Mark Allen, but we were working in an area where we had no idea what to do. However, taking this research further, after receiving some development funding for our quest to find a way to dissolve gallstones in the gallbladder and avoid surgery, we successfully constructed a gallbladder model.

The success of this new and innovative procedure, designed by me and my four fellow researchers, saw a paper published in 1981 in the top medical journal, the prestigious *New England Journal of Medicine*. I had a few papers published during my time at the Mayo, because I was also studying motility in the human gut and doing some in-vitro work on muscles, collecting ileum from dogs, which is the last section of the small intestine. This part of the bowel is important in several diseases, notably TB and Crohn's disease – a puzzle that would challenge me in the years to come.

The severe winter weather in Minnesota proved very difficult for my wife Sue and little Julie. Feeling claustrophobic, missing home, restless and unable to get out of the confines of our home, we all suffered 'cabin fever' and decided it was time to go home to Sydney. Looking back, this was a very important and influential time for me, my career and my connections. Indeed, it was a hell of an experience, being at the number one clinic in the world. I learnt how a major clinic works; I met the people whose names are in the textbooks; and my colleagues ended up as heads of their departments all over the world. It was an impressive place, and I was lucky to have the opportunity to go there. This experience inspired me to hope that, with luck and hard work, I too might make a valuable contribution to the advancement of medicine.

Chapter 1

Discovering the microbiome

From the rise of mankind, from the Neanderthals to the pharaohs of ancient Egypt, the human body and its diseases were a mystery. In classical Greece, Hippocrates, the 'Father of Medicine', was the first to classify diseases. He proposed that diseases were caused not by superstition or the Gods, but by an imbalance of four bodily fluids, something taken up by the Roman Aelius (or Claudius) Galenus, known to history as Galen. This established medicine as a separate profession, clear of philosophy and the practices and rituals of divine magic, which were the basis of medical beliefs at the time.

Apart from being the physician to Emperor Marcus Aurelius (161-180AD) Galen continued the work of Hippocrates, Aristotle and Plato, advancing what was known as the humoural theory. The four humours, blood, phlegm, black bile and yellow bile, would be the basis of medicine for the next 1,300 years. However, much like medical pioneers today, Galen's controversial teachings brought him into direct conflict with his contemporaries, who believed in mysticism and the inspiration of the Gods. This is perhaps the first example of how belief systems drive medical practice.

Galen was also interested in the gut and the whole gastrointestinal tract, starting at the mouth and finishing at the anus. He studied symptoms such as fever, vomiting, coughs, bad breath and severe ulceration of the trachea (windpipe) and the larynx (voice box) and other symptoms and ailments. He observed patients' stools and their diarrhea, noting that the blacker the stool, the sicker the person, with very black stools often preceding death. At this time, the dissection of a human cadaver was illegal, so he dissected animals in an effort to understand the human body. However, in the Middle Ages, physicians realised that the internal organs of animals were very different to humans. In fact, so influential was Galen's work that humourism and the belief in the four bodily fluids only ceased to be accepted medical theory with the arrival and understanding of germ theory. That is the understanding that many diseases are caused by microorganisms, pathogens or germs, which can only be observed under a microscope, an instrument not available to Galen.

Across the ancient world, parallel theories of human medicine were evolving. In China, the Taoist physicians were developing their own traditional medicines, including herbal preparations, massage, acupuncture and various other forms of therapy. Similarly in India, the medical belief of *Ayurveda*, 'the complete knowledge of long life' was codified in two definitive texts. In the Middle East, Islamic physicians and scientists developed the idea of hospitals and public health systems.

Back in Europe, by the thirteenth century, Galen's work was the basis of medical studies in all universities and was to remain so until a critical review of his theories by the Flemish physician and anatomist Andreas Vesalius (1514-1564), a colleague and housemate at Padua University of John Caius, who took the study of anatomy back to England. Vesalius began by dissecting human cadavers and comparing them with those of monkeys. He found many anatomical differences and concluded that Galen had only examined the corpses of apes. He went on to write some of the most important early books on human anatomy, *De Humani Corporis Fabrica Libri Septem* (*On the Fabric of the Human Body)* and came to be known as the 'father of human anatomy'.

Soon, other physicians began to discount Galen's theories, including the Italian Lazzaro Spallanzani (1729-1799) who studied the action of gastric acid in the stomach and showed that germs could be killed by boiling, thus providing fundamental research that later assisted Louis Pasteur. Others, like the German Philipp Bozzini (1773-1809), developed a primitive endoscope in 1807. This allowed an inspection of not only the urethra, the rectum, the bladder and the female cervix, but also the mouth, upper throat and ear. Primitive and limited though it was, this first endoscope allowed deeper and unseen internal parts of the living body to be studied and medically examined.

In 1823, a London-based physician and chemist named William Prout (1785-1850) took an interest in gut chemistry, which led him to discover that gastric juices contain hydrochloric acid, which he was able to separate by distillation. Four years later, he went on to identify various food substances as sugars, starch, oil and albumen, later to be reclassified as carbohydrates, fats and protein.

As the nineteenth century progressed, other physicians and researchers further extended knowledge of the gut and other vital organs in the stomach. However, there remained a major black spot in understanding disease transmission and the place of personal hygiene – germs. An Austrian, Ignaz Philipp Semmelweis (1818-1865) could not understand the high mortality of new mothers, where as many as 15% of them died from puerperal fever, also known as 'childbed fever'. In two obstetric wards, the first run by doctors and the second by mid-wives, he found that the death rate in the first ward was two to three times as high as that of the second – but why? The doctors of the time were proud to wear blood-covered gowns; the more blood, the more respected they were. They failed to realise that this blood contained the germs that caused the fever and the deaths. Semmelweis suggested doctors wash their hands and instruments prior to an operation. This was dismissed with contempt. His contemporaries were personally offended by his suggestion that they were the cause of the problem. Such was the ridicule he received, that he left the hospital and was committed to a mental asylum, where he died two weeks later, probably as a result of a savage beating by the guards.

This link between death and unhealthy procedures was taken up by a Frenchman, Louis Pasteur (1822-1895) a microbiologist and chemist who made several major medical breakthroughs, notably with 'pasteurisation', but also with vaccination and micro-bacterial fermentation. Meanwhile, an English-born surgeon and pathologist, Joseph Lister (1827-1912) was also doing groundbreaking medical research work, principally in Scotland, and became aware of Pasteur's work. Lister developed sterilisation procedures, using carbolic acid (known today as phenol) to prevent micro-organisms and germs entering the human body. This ensured sterile surgery, but he too was openly criticised by both the esteemed British Medical Journal, *The Lancet,* and the British Medical Association.

So, Lister, like Pasteur, moved the medical frontier forward yet again. Within 25 years, the use of carbolic acid and new surgical procedures in operating theatres brought about a dramatic drop in post-operative deaths. Lister was also the first surgeon to use catgut ligatures and sutures, the aortic tourniquet and a sterilised rubber tube as a drain.

In the nineteenth century, further research into the function of the gut was undertaken and new diseases were discovered. The problem was that various malignancies of the internal organs could not be seen and identified until they had reached an advanced stage or the patient died. The German Professor of Medicine, Adolf Kussmaul (1822-1902) first described dyslexia in 1877, attempted the first gastroscopy with what we know today as an endoscope, and performed gastric lavage to pump out the contents of the stomach. This work was again taken forward by Carl Stoerk (1832-1899) who specialised in remedial procedures of the throat, including an early endoscope device, which was quickly taken up and used to better understand and treat gut and intestinal problems with observation and diagnosis. In 1876, Karl Wilhelm von Kupffer (1829-1902), the Chair of Anatomy at Kiel University, wrote a paper describing the properties of cells he had studied in the liver, calling them Kupffer cells. These cells are the first line of defence for the liver.

The dawn of the twentieth century saw amazing advances in many areas of medicine and medical technology. Walter C. Alvarez (1884-1978), for example, undertook the first research into the electrical activity of the stomach in 1921-22. This opened the way for further research in what became electrogastrography. Another American chemist and physiologist, Jesse Francis McClendon (1880-1976) developed the first pH probe, that allowed the measurement of the gastric acid contents of the stomach *in situ*. All this research and exploration would benefit future researchers trying to understand the vast human microbiome, including my own work from the mid-1980s.

Throughout most of the twentieth century, gut microbes (including bacteria, viruses, and fungi) in the stool were considered either waste products or the culprits responsible for tissue infections. However, as research moved forward into the 21st century, we continue to shed this outdated notion. It is important to note that the first well-documented instance of a microbiome transplant, performed four times, took place in Colorado in 1957. I performed the first Faecal Microbiota Transplant (FMT) in Australia in 1988. By the middle of 1989, I had administered over fifty infusions and was often the first to provide a permanent cure for colitis in many of my patients.

There were rare instances of Scandinavian doctors also experimenting with the procedure at this time, but generally for indications in *Clostridioides difficile (C.difficile)* diarrhea. Primitive versions of microbiome therapy had already been used in traditional medicines in China and pioneered and documented in past scientific literature. Many of these findings lay dormant and unrecognised by the scientific community, overshadowed by the overpowering success of antibiotics.

As evidence of the importance of microbiomes in medicine mounted, a major research initiative called the Human Microbiome Project was begun in 2007, followed in 2014 with a re-launch of the project, using more advanced sequencing technologies to identify the bacterial species in the body. There were five major sites identified by the Human Microbiome Project, the nasal passages, oral cavity, skin, urogenital tract and the gut. However, despite remarkable advances in identifying thousands of commensal species of bacteria, scientists were still no closer to providing a molecular explanation of how microbiome transplantation cured the sick.

Microbiome-based medicine can be traced as far back as the tenth Century BC in China, where it was recorded that '*yellow soup*' was used to treat patients with infectious diseases. This was a concoction of fresh, dried or fermented faecal matter mixed with water and drunk by the patient to treat a range of abdominal conditions. The treatment was passed down in Chinese medicine and later documented in the fourth century AD by the Chinese doctor Ge Hong.

Accurate knowledge of microbiology was almost non-existent, but these treatments were effective enough to be continued for more than 2,600 years, until the sixteenth century. Interestingly, the method for administration always remained oral, with no exploration of enema-based practices. By chance, this pivotal discovery, administering faecal microbes by enema, remained unexplored for thousands of years. The Bedouins also are known to have used the fresh, even warm faeces of camels to treat bacterial dysentery, something taken up by the German Afrika Corps in the Second World War.

Discoveries relating to microbiology in western science would only emerge in the late seventeenth century. Even then, the full appreciation of microbes would not take off until much later. The Dutch scientist, Van Leeuwenhoek (1632-1723), developed his own microscopic lenses in 1681 and reported seeing 'animalcules' (small animals) in samples taken from his stools and teeth. Ultimately, these were called *Giardia lamblia*. Progress was slow. 150 years later, the German pathologist Friedrich Theodor von Frerichs (1819-1885) published extensively on his finding of harmless microorganisms living in the digestive tract.

By the end of the century, leading scientists from Britain, Germany and the United States would report similar findings of large numbers of bacteria in the stomach, intestines and stools, most of which could not be cultured. The belated finding that 'microbes are in our gut' seems somewhat ironic, given that the gut hosts the highest recorded density of microbes in any habitat on Earth. Only now have we come to grasp their presence and significance. For centuries, the scientific community resisted the study of our own microbiome, in favour of identifying bacteria everywhere else on Earth. Several more missed opportunities to explore the microbiome would ensue before we came closer to the truth of the microbiome's significance.

One major scientific milestone was reached in 1885 when the classification of stool bacteria in infants was investigated. The pathologist Theodor Escherich, (1857-1911) correctly identified that the bacteria of newborns transformed dramatically after birth. Escherich meticulously uncovered the role that many bacterial species had in an infant's diet as it shifted from breast milk to more solid foods. He was one of the first to cultivate and study bacterial species from the gut.

Escherich's work was quickly followed by Henri Tissier (1866-1952), a paediatrician at the Pasteur Institute in Paris, who believed that a particular bacterium could be given to new babies who had diarrhea, to replace pathogenic bacteria. He subsequently administered 'good bacteria' as a therapy to children with gastrointestinal diseases. With daily teaspoons of *Bacillus acidiparalactici*, he cured many children with diarrheal complaints. The success of his treatments led to similar treatment of adults with gastrointestinal disease, marking one of the earliest known probiotic treatments in western medicine.

Developments in the therapeutics of ingested bacteria, though a very small field, moved quickly, and in 1917, a prophylactic probiotic was developed against the backdrop of the First World War by the microbiologist Alfred Nissle (1874-1965). Nissle had been observing what he called 'bacterial antagonism', which occurred when stronger strains of intestinal microbes like *E.coli* could dominate and impede the growth of neighbouring pathogenic bacteria like Salmonella. Evidence for his theory was strengthened in the summer of 1917, when he observed a German corporal who had been deployed in operational areas on the Eastern Front, where deadly dysentery epidemics had occurred. Strangely, this corporal appeared to be immune to the disease, despite having constant contact with sick soldiers and consuming the same contaminated food and water as others around him. Nissle shrewdly suspected this soldier was carrying an antagonistically strong *E. coli* microbe that might have protected him from contracting dysentery, and had outcompeted other disease-causing microbes that he encountered. Nissle subsequently cultured the soldier's specific strain of bacteria in his laboratory and mass-produced *E.coli* in gelatine capsules. He successfully treated many soldiers and gave them immunity to dysentery with one of the first mass-produced and effective probiotic medicines. His invention was patented as a therapy with the name Mutaflor©, which continues to be sold to this day.

While many of these discoveries were revolutionary, they failed to challenge the prevailing belief that bacteria alone were responsible for disease. Many doctors and researchers disregarded their role as beneficial symbionts. This failure may have been due to the lack of sequencing technology at the time or the ignorance of probiotic species, which led many to discount the findings. Another factor that limited progress was poor understanding of the nature of anaerobic bacteria, which only grew under non-oxygenated conditions (not exposed to air). Subsequent studies showed that these anaerobic bacteria outnumbered aerobic bacteria by a thousand to one in the gut. These factors meant that for much of the twentieth century, little attention was paid to the microbiome, apart from the work of a few early pioneers.

Chapter 2

Seeing and studying the microbiome

Throughout history, medical practitioners could observe a patient's disease with the naked eye and provide their diagnosis on the basis of what was in front of them, but they could not enter the microscopic world that held the answer to diseases and the potential cures for them. Fortunately for us, the evolution of technologies, from culture-based methods and microscopy to advanced molecular techniques, next-generation sequencing and bioinformatics, has dramatically transformed our understanding of the human microbiome. These technological advances have enabled a more comprehensive and detailed exploration of the diversity, function and impact of microbial communities on human health.

As a result of this scientific innovation, our understanding of the human microbiome has significantly advanced over the past few decades. The earliest techniques were culture-based, where scientists relied on traditional microbiological techniques, such as culturing bacteria on nutrient media. These methods only identified a small fraction of the microbes that could grow under laboratory conditions. With these limitations, many microorganisms in the human body are unculturable under standard laboratory conditions, which limited our understanding of the full diversity of the microbiome.

The microbiome remained hidden, simply because the technology to view and study it was not available. Spectacles were invented in the fourteenth century and in 1590, a Dutch father and son team of spectacle makers (Hans and Zaccharias Janssen) built the first crude microscope. In 1667, the Dutch microbiologist, Anton van Leeuwenhoek (1632-1723) used a microscope to observe bacteria in rainwater. He called them animalcules, 'little animals'. He also made microscopic observations of red blood cells, crystals, spermatozoa and muscle fibres. He is generally regarded as the first true microbiologist.

Following this, microscopes became a necessary tool for medical researchers until 1981, when it became possible to get a three-dimensional image with the invention of the scanning, tunnelling microscope by Gerd Binnig and Heinrich Rohrer. Over this time, early observations of microorganisms using light microscopy provided basic insights into their presence and morphology. The electron microscope allowed for more detailed visualisation of microbial structures, but did not provide information on microbial diversity or function.

Today, many molecular technologies are available to revolutionise the study of the microbiome. For example, Polymerase Chain Reaction (PCR) has enabled the amplification of specific DNA sequences, allowing for the detection and identification of microbes without the need for culturing. Similarly, the 16S rRNA Gene Sequencing technique involves sequencing a conserved region of the bacterial 16S ribosomal RNA gene, allowing for the identification and classification of bacteria, which provides a more comprehensive view of bacterial diversity.

Metagenomics is also advancing our knowledge of the microbiome. This involves sequencing all the genetic material in a sample, providing a detailed and comprehensive view of the entire microbial community, including bacteria, archaea, viruses, fungi and other microorganisms. This approach can reveal not only the presence of different microbes, but also their potential functions. This provides a new and powerful way to understand the microbial environment and to reveal previously hidden and unknown microscopic life. Metagenomics also allows for the analysis of metabolic pathways and functional capabilities of microbial communities. It can even show us the unique composition of the microbiome in particular conditions, such as Parkinson's Disease.

Available today is Next-Generation Sequencing (NGS), high through-put sequencing technologies such as Illumina sequencing and nanopore sequencing, which have made it possible to sequence millions of DNA fragments simultaneously, greatly increasing the speed and reducing the cost of sequencing projects. Deep Sequencing allows for a more thorough and detailed analysis of microbial communities, including rare members. Then, by sequencing the RNA transcripts in a sample, scientists can study gene expression in microbial communities, providing insights into their active functions and interactions with the host.

Other technologies available to explore the microbiome include Proteomics, which involves the large-scale study of proteins produced by the microbiome, giving insights into the functional activity of microbial communities. Metabolomics or Metabolite Profiling studies the small molecules and metabolites produced by microbial communities, which can have significant effects on the host's physiology and health. Advanced bioinformatics tools and computational methods are essential for analysing the vast amounts of data generated by sequencing technologies. These tools help in identifying genes, assembling genomes and understanding the functional potential of microbial communities.

Microbiome archives have allowed the development of comprehensive databases for storing and comparing microbiome data from different studies and populations. Single cell genomics allows the study of individual microbial cells within a community, providing detailed insights into the diversity and functions of different microbial species. These technologies have brought about a significant increase in research, so that we now have a better understanding of the function, diversity and impact of microbial communities on our health and wellbeing.

Chapter 3

What is the microbiome?

Let us begin with a simple explanation.

The microbiome is the collection of all microorganisms including bacteria, archaea, fungi, viruses and other genetic material that live in and on the human body.

These microorganisms form complex communities and play crucial roles in human health and disease. Microbiomes also exist in the natural world, in animals, insects, the ocean and in the soil beneath our feet. There are believed to be 7.7 million different species of animals in the world, the majority being insects, arachnids, crustaceans and arthropods. By comparison, the number of species of microbes is estimated at one trillion, divided into seven types, bacteria, archaea, protozoa, algae, fungi, viruses, and multicellular animal parasites. Pick up a handful of rich soil and you will be holding a diverse community of billions of individual microorganisms, comprising tens of thousands of different species.

Soil microbiomes are essential for soil health and the functioning of healthy ecosystems. They play a crucial role in nutrient cycling, decomposition of organic matter, soil structure formation and plant growth. As in the human body, this important biodiversity is seriously threatened by comparatively recent developments: microbe communities in the soil are in serious decline due to the effects of various synthetic chemicals on the natural biome.

In our body, there is a vast, unknown and barely researched world of microbiota. While estimates vary, it is believed there are more than 1,000 species of microbes at home in our colon. Just one gram of human 'poo' contains perhaps 100 billion bacteria. It is indeed a hectic yet industrious micro-environment. Here the microbiome manifests itself by forming complex communities of microorganisms that reside in various 'suburbs' of our bodies including the skin, the mouth and the respiratory, gastrointestinal and urogenital tracts. The composition of the microbiomes of these organs can vary considerably. These microorganisms play an essential role in maintaining our health by aiding digestion, protecting against pathogens and modulating the immune system.

Our microbiome begins as a gift from our mother. During a vaginal birth, the baby passes through the birth canal, where it is exposed to and provided with the complete range of the mother's microbiota. In this way, key bacteria such as the natural probiotic *Lactobacillus*, and *Bifidobacterium*, an anaerobic bacterium which boosts immunity, are transferred to the newborn, colonising the skin, mouth and gut. These early microbial exposures help to stimulate the baby's immune system and establish a healthy microbiome.

This gift continues after the birth, first by skin-to-skin contact where further colonisation occurs and with breast feeding, where maternal antibodies and microbia are also transferred. The very first flush of breast milk - colostrum, is high in protein, vitamins, minerals, nutrient-rich and high also in antibodies and antioxidants, crucial in establishing a newborn baby's immune system. Containing beneficial bacteria and probiotics, it promotes the growth of a healthy gut microbiome in the infant – a very important start to life.

The importance of this maternal microbiome can be seen in a number of areas. With digestive health, it establishes a robust and balanced gut microbiome in the newborn, crucial for digestion and nutrient absorption. For the immune system, early exposure to maternal microbiomes primes the infant's immune system, reducing the risk of allergies, asthma and other immune-related conditions. It also provides protection against pathogens, as a well-established microbiome offers a defence against pathogenic microorganisms by out-competing them and modulating the infant's immune responses.

So, the maternal microbiome plays a pivotal role in shaping our future, starting with the infant's microbiome during vaginal birth, significantly influencing the child's health by aiding in the development of the immune system, digestion and protection against pathogens. This foundational microbial exposure sets the stage for lifelong health and wellbeing. However, it is interesting to note that while the mother provides her newborn with 100 percent of her microbiome, the father may also add to the mix. It has been found that long-established cohabiting couples develop a broadly complementary microbiome, so the father also contributes indirectly to the newborn's microbiome and wellbeing.

In trying to understand the microbiome, let us look at where it is found in the human body and where it is distributed. In the skin, microbes are found in bacteria, fungi and viruses. Their function is to protect against pathogens, contribute to the immune system and maintain skin health. There are several common genera: *Staphylococcus*, commonly known as staph infections, are found on the skin and in the nose in many healthy people, but only become dangerous if they enter the body through the bloodstream and infect the heart, lungs or other organs. *Corynebacterium* is widely distributed in nature; while mostly innocuous, it is the cause of diphtheria. *Propionibacterium* is found in the skin, hair and the gastrointestinal tract.

In the mouth, there are also microbiota in the form of bacteria, fungi and viruses. Their role is to begin the digestion process, prevent colonisation by pathogens and maintain good oral health. Here again we find *Streptococcus* but also *Neisseria*, the most common cause of bacterial meningitis in children and *Veillonella*, an anaerobic bacterium that can cause tooth decay and gum disease.

In the respiratory tract there are bacteria and fungi which work to protect against pathogens and maintain respiratory health. Along with *Streptococcus* there is *Haemophilus*, a serious bacterial disease that can lead to a potentially deadly brain infection and may cause meningitis, particularly among young children. Also found in the respiratory tract is *Moraxella* which can cause ear and sinus infections, particularly in children, and can cause meningitis and pneumonia in adults.

In the urogenital tract we have the same three, bacteria, fungi and viruses, which work to protect against infections and maintain urinary and reproductive health. Here the common genera are first *Lactobacillus,* mentioned above, but also *Gardnerella*, a bacterium in the vagina to keep it free of infection, and *Prevotella,* believed to assist in keeping blood sugar levels in a safe range, which can protect against cardiovascular diseases. However, there is conflicting research which suggests it can lead to hypertension, obesity, bowel disease and other ailments.

Finally, in the gastrointestinal tract, we find the same bacteria, whose job there is to assist digestion, nutrient absorption, strengthen the immune function and provide protection against pathogens. Here we also find the common genera, *Bacteroides, Firmicutes* plus *Lactobacillus* and *Bifidobacterium,* as mentioned above. *Bacteroides* is an intestinal bacterium which exists with the host in a beneficial relationship, but when it escapes the gut, it can cause bacteraemia and the formation of abscesses. Abnormal *Firmicutes* may contribute to many diseases including heart problems, some cancers, Type 1 and Type 2 diabetes, gastrointestinal disfunction and even obesity. This is the largest storehouse of microbiome, particularly in the colon, and contains the highest density and diversity of microorganisms in the body, playing vital roles in digestion, metabolism, and immune regulation.

Billions of bacteria make up the human microbiome; these are but a few of the key ones. It is important to remember that it is not only the genera, but also the numbers of specific genera that matter. The balance is crucial; you cannot have just one kind of 'good' bacteria: you need a community, as a healthy microbiome is dependent upon diversity, mutual reliance and symbiosis.

The microbiome is crucial for life, because it plays several vital roles in maintaining human health and well-being. In digestive health, the microbiome helps break down complex carbohydrates, proteins and fats, aiding in nutrient absorption and energy production. It also assists vitamin synthesis, as certain bacteria produce essential vitamins such as vitamin K and some B vitamins. Another important function is ensuring immunity: the microbiome helps to train and modulate the immune system, cleverly deciding between harmful and harmless substances while working to out-compete pathogenic organisms by providing a protective barrier against infection.

Another critical role our microbiome plays in maintaining health and wellbeing is in our metabolic function, the chemical process that breaks down nutrients by converting food and drink into the energy we need to build and repair our bodies. In this regard, our microbial communities influence metabolic processing, which in turn affects our body weight and works to prevent metabolic diseases like diabetes. They also help gut bacteria to ferment indigestible fibres, producing short-chain fatty acids that nourish gut cells and regulate inflammation.

In a world of rapidly transmittable diseases and pandemics, our microbiome plays a crucial role in protecting us against illness. First, by preventing infection, a healthy microbiome prevents colonisation by potentially dangerous pathogens: it occupies niches within our bodies and produces antimicrobial substances as a form of defence. Our microbiome also helps to control inflammatory responses, reducing the risk of chronic infections.

Our microbiota also play an important part in our mental health. Recent research has found there is a two-way communication between the gut and the brain, something known as the 'gut-brain axis' (GBA). Within this, our microbiome influences brain function, linking gut problems with certain nervous disorders, such as autism, anxiety, depressive behaviours and bi-polar conditions. This might sound surprising, but we are also learning that gastrointestinal disorders like irritable bowel syndrome may be the result of a disruption in this complex gut-brain communication system where there is abnormality in the microbiome.

It is not surprising that the skin of our bodies, in fact our largest organ, is the home to a diverse community of microorganisms. Most are harmless; many are beneficial. Skin microbiota are very diverse and variable: they help to maintain the skin barrier, protect against pathogens, modulate skin immunity, and educate our immune system. A balanced skin microbiome reduces the risk of conditions like eczema and acne.

Our microbiome also affects our reproductive health. The vagina provides a warm, humid and nutritious host environment to billions of microbes. While the microbiota of our respiratory and intestinal systems have long been the focus of research attention, reproductive health has received far less interest until recently. With an increasing emphasis on female health, attention has been drawn to the vaginal microbiome, where the dominant species, *Lactobacillus* maintains a low pH environment to protect women against infections and support reproductive health.

Finally, the microbiome is vital to our respiratory health. Just like the gut-brain axis, the gut-lung axis forms a bi-directional, symbiotic relationship between the lungs and the gut. This communication, mediated by the microbiome, influences immune responses, inflammation and overall health in both organs. The microbiome contained in the lung is directly linked to various chronic lung diseases like asthma, lung cancer and chronic obstructive pulmonary disease.

Our microbiome, therefore, is integral to numerous physiological processes that are essential for maintaining good health. It aids digestion, nutrient synthesis, immune regulation, metabolic function, disease prevention, mental health, skin health and reproductive health. Disruptions in the microbiome can lead to a multitude of health issues, highlighting its importance for life.

Chapter 4

The microbiome under attack

The importance of maintaining a healthy and balanced microbiome is the great challenge of medicine today. When our microbiome becomes infected, often with unculturable pathogens, it is called 'dysbiotic'. Dysbiosis is an imbalance in the microbial communities, particularly of the gut, where the normal composition and function of the microbiota are disrupted. This disturbance can lead to various health problems, as the gut microbiota plays a critical role in digestion, immune function, and overall health. Other contributors to gut dysbiosis include antibiotic use, poor diet, stress, infections and various lifestyle and environmental factors. Maintaining healthy and balanced gut microbiota is crucial for preventing these health issues.

What are the major contributors to gut dysbiosis and what are the consequences?

First, we have antibiotics. We all know how important antibiotics have proved to be, since the first application of Penicillin in the early 1940s. Each year, antibiotics save millions of lives around the world, but unfortunately, by taking antibiotics, you disrupt the very complex matrix of ecosystems that make up your human microbiome. Broad-spectrum antibiotics can kill both pathogenic and beneficial bacteria, leading to a reduction in microbial diversity and an overgrowth by resistant or opportunistic pathogens. Add to this antibiotic resistance and we have the making of a severe global health problem which could affect us all. Here we see reduced microbial diversity, along with other damaging attributes, making individuals more susceptible to infection by pathogens like the gut bacteria *Clostridioides difficile.*

Second, we have diet. As we all know, the aggressive advertising of the fast-food outlets and the processed food industries encourage dietary choices that can alter the gut microbiome. This can lead to widespread obesity, heart disease, stroke and type 2 diabetes, but do people think about what they are putting into their gut? Do they realise that the more you process food and include additives, the further you remove it from its nutritious natural state, so that less nutritional value is retained? Processed foods are often high in sugar, salt, fats and other synthetic additives and presented ready to eat in striking packaging, making them attractive to less health-conscious people. This nutritionally unbalanced diet, often with a long shelf life, thanks to preservatives, is regrettably responsible for much of the obesity and the related disease crises of today.

It is clear that a high intake of processed foods, sugar and unhealthy fats has a negative impact upon our gut microbiota. Combined with a shortage of dietary fibre, this causes a reduction in the production of short-chain fatty acids (SCFAs) which play an important part in maintaining good health and fighting disease. This helps to explain the increased prevalence of a range of inflammatory diseases, particularly in wealthy Western countries, where considerations of convenience, taste and price persuade consumers to replace a balanced, natural diet. We should always look for variety and a natural alternative, such as fresh fruit and vegetables, nuts and wholegrain rice and oats.

Third, we must consider infection. In this regard, pathogenic infections, whether bacterial, viral or parasitic, can disrupt the balance of the gut microbiota by introducing harmful microorganisms that outcompete beneficial ones and can secrete various toxins. Within our gut microbiome, parasites occupy the same environment as bacteria and so can cause an imbalance in our normal, healthy gut microbiota. This can result in diarrhea and colitis, with some infections attacking the gut lining and gaining access to the bloodstream. This leads to dysbiosis, which in turn weakens the gut's ability to defend itself against these same, harmful pathogens.

Fourth, we have the effects of stress. While we all experience stress, either mental or physical, we may not see a link between our brain's stress response and our gut microbiota. Yet our daily gastrointestinal function is particularly influenced by the stresses we endure. The most common adverse conditions are diarrhea, constipation, heartburn, vomiting and lower abdominal pain. Psychological stress can alter gut motility, permeability and the production of mucus, which in turn affects the composition of the gut microbiota.

Fifth, while we have seen the effect antibiotics can have on our gut microbiota, we must also consider the effects of non-antibiotic medications. Research has shown that certain medications, including proton pump inhibitors, medications which reduce stomach acid, non-steroidal anti-inflammatory drugs (NSAIDs) and others, can all affect the gut microbiota. NSAIDs are the most commonly used drugs worldwide, because they alleviate both inflammation and pain in arthritis and other musculoskeletal diseases, but in the process, they can damage the stomach and intestine and alter the gut microbiota. Studies have also found a strong correlation between popular medications like statins, metformin and opioids on gut microbiota signatures.

Sixth, lifestyle and environmental factors can also affect our gut microbiota. Lack of a good night's sleep and poor sleep patterns can disrupt the circadian rhythms of gut bacteria. So can a sedentary lifestyle. The absence of physical activity is often associated with an unfavourable gut microbiota composition. Similarly, environmental factors can directly affect our microbiota and hence our health. Exposure to environmental toxins and pollutants can negatively impact the gut microbiota, while the overuse of sanitisers and antiseptics can reduce our exposure to beneficial microbes. Even exposure to sunlight has been found to be beneficial. Some research has noted the negative effects of blue light, which can have health issues and unexpected consequences.

Seventh, we must include our medical conditions and any chronic diseases we have. An imbalance of the normal gut microbiota has been associated with gastrointestinal conditions like irritable bowel syndrome (IBS) and inflammatory bowel disease (IBD) along with obesity, type 2 diabetes and atopy, the medical condition whereby your immune system makes you more likely to contact and develop allergic diseases. Dysbiosis can therefore be both the cause and the consequence of autoimmune illness. Chronic diseases are also associated with dysbiosis, making them another contributory factor that can impact your gut microbiota.

An eighth cause is age and genetics. The natural aging process can lead to changes in the gut microbiota composition and function. In young men, the gut microbiome often has a diverse and balanced composition. *Firmicutes* and *Bacteroides* are two of the major phyla, but their relative abundance can vary widely among individuals. Studies have suggested that, as people age, there can be a decrease in microbial diversity and changes in the relative abundances of different bacterial groups. Some research indicates an increase in *Bacteroides* and a decrease in *Firmicutes*, but this is not universally true. Research has also shown a gradual increase in bacterial richness as people age and a corresponding and gradual decrease in bacterial diversity. This re-balance of gut bacteria is a crucial factor, affecting inflammation, immunity and the development of disease.

So, what are the consequences of gut dysbiosis?

A dysbiotic microbiome has been associated with symptoms like bloating, diarrhea, constipation and irritable bowel syndrome. There is increased risk of intestinal permeability, also known as 'leaky gut', which in turn can lead to systemic inflammation and contribute to conditions like IBS. There are also metabolic disorders, where dysbiosis is linked to obesity, insulin resistance and type 2 diabetes, while imbalanced gut microbiota can affect the immune system, increasing an individual's susceptibility to infections and autoimmune diseases. Dysbiosis is also associated with mental health issues like anxiety, depression and cognitive decline, through the gut-brain axis.

It is important, for a healthy and disease-free lifestyle, to maintain a healthy and balanced microbiome. As we have seen, when our gut microbiota are disturbed, for example by a pathogen, we may develop a dysbiotic microbiome. This is a negative for our health and a sign to change whatever it is that is causing the condition.

Pathogens can have a profound impact on the gut microbiome by disrupting the balance of microbial communities, triggering inflammation, altering the gut environment and competing for nutrients. These changes can lead to a range of health issues, both within the gut and systemically. The major impact of a pathogen in the gut microbiome can cause alterations in the composition and function of the microbial community. When there is a disruption in the microbial balance, we see a reduction in beneficial bacteria, such as *Lactobacillus* and *Bifidobacterium*, which are crucial for maintaining gut health. The presence of a pathogen can lead to its overgrowth and dominance, further disrupting the balance of the gut microbiota.

Also affected are our inflammation and immune responses. Pathogens can trigger an immune response, leading to inflammation in the gut, which can damage the gut lining and alter the habitat of the gut microbiota. In turn, the immune system's efforts to combat the pathogen can also affect the resident microbiota, potentially leading to long-term changes in microbial composition. Similarly, changes in pathogens can alter the pH of the gut, making it less hospitable for certain beneficial microbes and more conducive to the growth of other pathogens. Along with this, some pathogens produce toxins that can damage gut tissue and disrupt the microbial ecosystem.

Then there is the issue of nutrient competition. Pathogens may compete with beneficial microbes for nutrients, depriving them of the essential resources they need for their growth and function. Infections can increase gut permeability, allowing pathogens, toxins and partially digested food particles to enter the bloodstream, which can cause systemic inflammation and affect distant organs.

There are also secondary infections to consider. The disruption caused by a primary pathogen can create opportunities for secondary infections by other pathogens, further complicating the gut microbial balance and seriously affecting your health. This can have an impact on your metabolism: pathogen-induced dysbiosis can affect the metabolic activities of the gut microbiota, leading to changes in the production of short-chain fatty acids and other metabolites that are important for gut health.

We should not forget the long-term health effects. Persistent dysbiosis caused by pathogens can contribute to the development of chronic gastrointestinal conditions, such as inflammatory bowel disease (IBD) and irritable bowel syndrome (IBS) as mentioned above. And with systemic effects, the impact of gut pathogens can extend beyond the gut, potentially influencing conditions like metabolic syndrome, obesity and even mental health disorders, through the gut-brain axis.

Chapter 5

The microbiome's defence

So, what defence mechanisms does our microbiome have?

Fortunately, it has multiple defence mechanisms to protect human health, which can prevent pathogenic colonisation, modulate the immune system, strengthen the gut barrier, support metabolic functions, detoxify harmful compounds and regulate inflammation. These mechanisms singly and collectively contribute to maintaining overall health and preventing disease.

By resisting colonisation and excluding competition, beneficial microbes occupy niches and utilise available nutrients, preventing pathogenic organisms from implanting and proliferating. Along with this, many commensal bacteria, that is non-pathogenic inhabitants of the microbiome, produce substances such as bacteriocins, short-chain fatty acids (SCFAs) and other antimicrobial peptides that inhibit the growth of pathogens. By training the immune system, the microbiome helps to educate and regulate the immune response. It teaches it to differentiate between harmful and harmless entities, which is indeed an amazing capability. By enhanced immune responses, commensal bacteria stimulate the production of antibodies and activate immune cells, enhancing the ability to fight infections throughout the body and restore a healthy microbiome.

The microbiome's defence mechanisms also function as a barrier, by strengthening the gut lining. Here, beneficial microbes promote the integrity of the gut epithelial barrier by stimulating the production of mucus and tight junction proteins, which help prevent pathogens and toxins from entering the bloodstream. It also provides mucosal protection whereby the mucus layer, produced by goblet cells in the gut, traps pathogens. The mucus contains antimicrobial proteins that neutralise the pathogens.

Meanwhile, SCFAs, produced by the fermentation of dietary fibres by gut bacteria (such as acetate, propionate, and butyrate) have anti-inflammatory properties and provide energy to gut epithelial cells, again promoting gut health. Gut microbes also synthesise essential nutrients, including certain vitamins (e.g. vitamin K and B vitamins), that support overall health and immune function. Through the degradation of harmful compounds, the microbiome can metabolise and neutralise potential toxins, including dietary toxins and environmental pollutants, reducing their harmful effects on the body.

Another of the microbiome's defence mechanisms is regulating inflammation. Beneficial microbes help maintain a balanced inflammatory response, preventing excessive inflammation, which can damage tissues and lead to complications. They also support the gut-brain axis: the gut bacteria produce neurotransmitters, such as serotonin and gamma-aminobutyric acid (GABA), which influence brain function and mood. They help to avoid symptoms like 'foggy brain', slow thinking and vagueness, often associated with chronic fatigue. A healthy microbiome is also associated with a reduced risk of mental health issues, such as depression and anxiety, acting through the gut-brain axis.

As we have seen, the gut-lung axis refers to the intricate relationship between the gut microbiome and the respiratory system. This two-way communication involves microbial influence on systemic immune responses, impacting inflammation and immune reactions in the lungs. Metabolites produced by gut bacteria, such as SCFAs, can reach the lungs via the bloodstream and affect local immune responses. Additionally, a healthy gut microbiome plays a crucial role in maintaining gut barrier integrity, which reduces systemic inflammation, which could potentially impact lung health.

Chapter 6

The microbiome recovers

How do these defence mechanisms work and how long does recovery take?

A healthy microbiome defends itself against pathogenic invasion through competitive exclusion, production of antimicrobial substances, modulation of immune responses, enhancement of gut barrier function, metabolic interference and resistance to colonisation. These defence mechanisms collectively help to maintain microbial balance and protect against infections, supporting overall gut health and host immunity.

The principle of competitive exclusion, sometimes referred to as Gause's law, states that when two species, or in this case two bacteria, compete for the same resources, then one species will dominate, causing either the extinction of the other or else making it shift to another niche. In this case, a healthy microbiome employs several defence mechanisms to protect itself from invasion by pathogens: it allows beneficial microbes to occupy ecological niches in the gut, where they compete with pathogens for space and nutrients. Similarly, through resource competition, the beneficial microbes outcompete pathogens by consuming available resources, limiting the growth and establishment of pathogenic species.

Through the production of antimicrobial substances, our beneficial bacteria produce bacteriocins, which are antimicrobial peptides that inhibit the growth of pathogens. They are anti-inflammatory and assist digestion and the use of energy in our bodies. Also, some microbes produce metabolites like SCFAs that create an acidic environment unfavourable for pathogens. They assist in the modulation of the immune response, as commensal bacteria help to educate and regulate the immune system, training it to recognise and respond appropriately to pathogens. They also promote a balanced immune response, reducing excessive inflammation, which can result in colitis or Crohn's disease, which would harm both the microbiome and the host.

As part of this defence, beneficial bacteria enhance the gut barrier function by stimulating mucus production by intestinal epithelial cells. These form a physical barrier that prevents pathogens from adhering to and penetrating the gut lining. They also support the integrity of tight junctions between epithelial cells, maintaining gut barrier function and preventing the translocation of pathogens across the intestinal barrier into other parts of the body. Also, by indirect pathogen inhibition, beneficial microbes metabolise nutrients in a way that interferes with the growth and survival of pathogens and can neutralise toxins produced by them, reducing their harmful effects on the gut environment. Finally, a diverse and healthy microbiome can resist colonisation by pathogens simply by occupying available niches and maintaining microbial diversity.

The recovery of the gut microbiome after a pathogenic invasion involves a process of immune response, clearance of pathogens, repopulation by resilient microbes, restoration of diversity and the modulation of immune function. The duration of this recovery can vary widely and is influenced by multiple factors, emphasising the importance of supporting gut health through balanced nutrition and probiotic/prebiotic interventions. After a pathogenic invasion disrupts the gut microbiome, the recovery process typically involves several stages, and the timeline can vary, depending on factors such as the severity of the infection, the individual's overall health and the specific pathogens involved. Let us observe how the gut microbiome recovers.

In simple terms, when we eat a meal, we consume vast numbers of microbes, including bacteria and fungi. During its passage through the acidic stomach, the bacterial load is diminished. When bathed in bile and pancreatic enzymes, there is further reduction in bacterial numbers. These zones are the body's natural filters to remove pathogens. However, some remaining organisms enter the small bowel and ultimately the colon, where further clearance of pathogens occurs. This is achieved by commensal bacteria, which eradicate most of the pathogens.

Then, to remove any remaining pathogens, antibiotics can be used, or other treatments such as faecal microbiota transplant (FMT) can directly target and eliminate these pathogens, after which there is repopulation by resilient microbes. These resilient species are beneficial bacteria that survived the initial disturbance and now begin to proliferate and restore microbial diversity. The recovery process also involves these resilient microbes re-establishing their populations and competing with potential pathogens for niche space. Over time, microbial diversity gradually returns to a healthier state, as more species re-colonise the gut and different species resume their roles in supporting digestion, nutrient metabolism and immune regulation.

To further assist recovery, the immune system begins rebalancing with the gut microbiome, helping to regulate immune responses, by promoting a balanced environment that supports ongoing recovery and prevents further infections. The recovery timeline can range from days to weeks or even longer, depending on factors such as the type of pathogen, the extent of damage to the microbiome and individual health conditions. Each person's microbiome recovery process will differ according to their immune system resilience, diet, lifestyle and medical history. Nonetheless, despite all these efficient mechanisms, some pathogens, such as *Clostridiodes difficile*, remain difficult to eradicate.

Finally, the factors affecting recovery include antibiotic use, the consumption of both probiotics and prebiotics and dietary changes. If antibiotics have been used to treat the infection, they may disrupt the microbiome further and extend the recovery time. The consumption of probiotics (beneficial bacteria) and prebiotics (fibre that promotes the growth of beneficial bacteria) can support faster recovery. Meanwhile, a balanced diet, rich in fibre and nutrients, supports microbial diversity and promotes gut health.

How can medicines and drugs assist this recovery?

Medicines and drugs play crucial roles in supporting microbiome recovery. They do this by introducing beneficial bacteria (probiotics), providing nutrients for their growth (prebiotics), restoring microbial diversity (FMT) and judiciously managing antibiotic use. These approaches help to mitigate the impact of disruptions to the microbiome and promote gut health, thereby supporting overall well-being and immune function. Medicines and drugs can assist in the recovery of the microbiome in several ways, particularly after disruption caused by infections, antibiotics or other factors.

Let us look at these in order. First, probiotics introduce beneficial bacteria. Probiotics are live microorganisms that, when administered in adequate amounts, confer health benefits on the host. They can help replenish and diversify the gut microbiota, especially after antibiotic treatment or pathogenic infections. Probiotics such as *Lactobacillus* and *Bifidobacterium* species can enhance gut barrier function, modulate immune responses and compete with pathogens for colonisation sites. Secondly, prebiotics provide fuel for beneficial bacteria. These prebiotics are dietary fibres that selectively stimulate the growth and activity of beneficial bacteria already present in the gut. By promoting the growth of beneficial microbes, prebiotics contribute to the restoration of microbial diversity and ecosystem stability.

A proven process to assist the recovery of gut microbiota is via Faecal Microbiota Transplantation (FMT). This medical process involves transferring faecal material from a healthy donor to a recipient to restore balanced gut microbiota and cure an infective condition. It has been particularly successful in treating recurrent *Clostridium difficile* infections and is being researched for other conditions where microbiome restoration has been found to be beneficial.

An important aspect of antimicrobial use is antibiotic stewardship. By preserving microbial diversity through careful and proper antibiotic use, (including targeted and narrow-spectrum antibiotics), this minimises disruption to the gut microbiome. Also, by a combination of therapies and proper antibiotic use, including targeted and narrow-spectrum antibiotics that preserve microbial diversity, there is minimal disruption to the gut microbiome. Meanwhile, some antibiotics are designed to target specific pathogens with minimal impact on beneficial gut bacteria.

To further assist recovery, there are microbiome-modulating drugs which are an emerging therapy with the aim of selectively modulating the gut microbiota to promote health. These include bacteriophages (viruses that target specific bacteria) and other microbiome-targeted therapeutics which are in development. There are also lifestyle and dietary interventions and emerging therapies which support microbial health. Adopting a diet rich in fibre, fermented foods and nutrients supports the growth of beneficial gut bacteria. Lifestyle factors such as regular exercise and adequate sleep also contribute to maintaining a healthy microbiome.

However, drugs can also damage and affect the human microbiome in several negative ways. Antibiotics are designed to kill or inhibit the growth of bacteria, but they can disrupt not only the target pathogens, but also beneficial bacteria in the gut. Prolonged or frequent antibiotic use can lead to a reduction in microbial diversity, making the gut more susceptible to colonisation by opportunistic pathogens. Unfortunately, the overuse of antibiotics can promote the development of antibiotic-resistant strains of bacteria, which may persist in the gut microbiome.

Non-antibiotic medications can also have negative effects on the human microbiome. Medications such as proton pump inhibitors (PPIs), non-steroidal anti-inflammatory drugs (NSAIDs) and certain antidepressants can alter the composition and function of the gut microbiota. Some drugs may affect microbial metabolism, potentially leading to shifts in the production of metabolites that influence gut and overall health.

Similarly, cancer treatments like chemotherapy and immunosuppressive drugs can directly impact gut bacteria due to their cytotoxic effects. These immune system suppression drugs can compromise the body's ability to regulate and maintain a healthy microbiome. Some drugs can increase intestinal permeability, known as 'leaky gut'. This allows harmful substances and pathogens to enter the bloodstream and affect systemic health. Gut dysbiosis induced by drugs can also trigger inflammatory responses in the gut.

Changes in the composition of the gut microbiota can affect the metabolism and absorption of nutrients essential for overall health, further damaging the microbiome. Vitamin deficiencies can occur, as some medications may interfere with the gut microbiota's ability to produce natural vitamins. This raises the risk of chronic diseases and presents long-term implications. Disruption of the gut microbiome by drugs has been linked to an increased risk of chronic conditions such as obesity, metabolic syndrome and autoimmune diseases. Microbial resistance, like antibiotic resistance, can also arise with the misuse or overuse of medications. Resistance in the gut microbiota can compromise or complicate future treatments.

Is the damage from viral or bacterial attacks permanent or can the microbiome recover completely?

While the microbiome has a remarkable capacity for recovery after bacterial or viral attacks, the process and extent of recovery can vary. With appropriate support and interventions, including probiotics, dietary adjustments and immune system management, the microbiome can often restore balance and functionality over time. However, severe or chronic infections may leave lasting impacts, underscoring the importance of proactive management and health monitoring in maintaining gut health and overall well-being.

Chapter 7

Other microbiome communities in nature

As explained, our bodies contain a number of different microbiome communities. They can be found in our gut, on our skin and down our respiratory tract. This microbiome diversity is not restricted to humans, but can be found throughout nature – in animals, insects, the ocean and in the soil beneath our feet.

Microbial diversity is crucial in plant growth, in nutrient cycling, in decomposition within living organisms and in soil structure formation. While there are similarities in microbial functions and interactions across species, human and animal microbiomes differ significantly in composition, diversity, ecological adaptations and geographical disposition. These differences reflect unique evolutionary paths, dietary habits, environmental exposures and host-microbe interactions, highlighting the complexity and variety of microbial ecosystems across the animal kingdom. For example, human gut microbiomes typically include *Firmicutes, Bacteroidetes, Actinobacteria* and *Proteobacteria*, whereas cows and other animals have specialised microbes (e.g., *Ruminococcus*) for cellulose digestion. Animal gut microbiomes often contain enzymes and metabolic pathways adapted for digesting complex plant or animal materials or facilitating nutrient absorption from specialised diets.

Soil has its own microbiome, in which we find a diverse community of micro-organisms, including bacteria, fungi, archaea, viruses and other microbes. Soil microbiomes are essential for soil health and ecosystem functioning, playing crucial roles in nutrient cycling, decomposition of organic matter, soil structure formation and plant growth. When we explore the composition of the soil microbiome, we find that the dominant bacterial phyla in soil include *Proteobacteria, Actinobacteria, Firmicutes* and *Bacteroidetes*. These bacteria contribute to nutrient cycling by decomposing organic matter and fixing nitrogen.

Also present in the soil microbiota are fungi, archaea and viruses. Soil fungi include both saprotrophs (which decompose organic matter) and mycorrhizal fungi which form symbiotic relationships with plant roots, aiding in nutrient uptake. *Archaea* in soil often play a role in nutrient cycling processes such as nitrification and methane oxidation. In the case of soil viruses, or bacteriophages, they work to infect and control bacterial populations, thereby influencing the dynamics within microbial communities. In short, everything has its own microbiome, including air, water (the marine microbiome is different from the freshwater microbiome) and the earth below us.

What is the importance of this to life on earth as we know it? And is there a crossover between the soil/earth microbiome and the human/animal microbiome?

The microbiomes of sea, air, water and soil all interact with the human microbiome in intricate ways essential for ecological balance and human health. Marine microbiomes contribute to global nutrient cycling and climate regulation, influencing the composition of atmospheric gases and providing essential nutrients for seafood consumption. Soil microbiomes support agriculture by enhancing soil fertility and nutrient availability, determining the quality of crops and food. Airborne microbiomes influence human health through respiratory exposure, potentially affecting immune responses and respiratory conditions. Water microbiomes, including those in freshwater and marine environments, affect drinking water quality and aquatic biodiversity, influencing human health directly through waterborne diseases and indirectly through food chains. Understanding these interactions is crucial for managing environmental health. We need to promote sustainable practices and maintain the diversity and resilience of both natural ecosystems and human microbiomes.

Within this diverse and extensive world of varying microbiomes, is the human microbiome evolving, in response to new threats, drugs and diseases?

As one might expect, the human microbiome continues to evolve, especially when faced with these new challenges. Key aspects of its ongoing evolution include the need to adapt to modern environments, to respond to medical interventions, and to confront emerging diseases and pathogens. It must maintain its genetic and functional diversity and the potential for therapeutic innovations. As human lifestyles and environments change, so does the microbiome. Over time, diet, sanitation practices, exercise, antibiotic use and exposure to pollutants can and do alter the composition and diversity of the microbiome.

The microbiome can respond to medical intervention. This is especially the case with antibiotics, chemotherapy and other medications, which can selectively impact the microbiome, leading to compositional shifts in microbial communities and potential adaptations to these treatments. Parallel to this, the microbiome faces new challenges from emerging infectious diseases and pathogens. Host-microbe interactions evolve as microbes adapt to defend against or exploit these threats, influencing disease susceptibility and immune responses.

In today's world, the microbiome must also respond to environmental factors. These include climate change, pollution and urbanisation, which can affect microbial diversity and community structure, potentially influencing human health outcomes and ultimately mortality. The human microbiome must also address genetic and functional diversity. Variability in human genetic backgrounds and microbial genomes contributes to the diversity of microbiome compositions observed across populations. Microbial functions and metabolic capabilities can evolve in response to selective pressures imposed by host immune systems and environmental factors.

Given all of this, we must actively spread the word on the importance of the human microbiome in our health and wellbeing and persuade people to respect and value these crucial elements within our bodies. Popularising the human microbiome story and fostering an understanding of its importance can be achieved in several ways: we could launch educational campaigns in schools, community centres and online platforms, to raise awareness about the microbiome's role in health and disease; we could collaborate with media outlets to feature stories, documentaries and articles that highlight the microbiome's significance and its impact on everyday life.

Given its growing importance, education should be integrated with health care practices and training, where healthcare professionals learn about the microbiome's influence on health outcomes, emphasising its role in digestion, immunity and disease prevention. Taking this further, there should be means to equip patients with information on how lifestyle choices, diet and medications affect their microbiome. This process would empower them to make more informed decisions.

Spreading the net further, we could include community engagement and participation. This might include organising public events, workshops and seminars, where experts discuss the microbiome's importance and answer community questions. We might also consider citizen science initiatives to engage the public in microbiome research through projects that allow individuals to contribute samples or participate in data collection. Similarly, we could showcase microbiome-themed art exhibitions, performances and literature to explore the intersection of science and creativity, making the topic accessible and engaging. To highlight the connection between diet, gut health and human microbiome diversity, we could extend community involvement through cooking classes, food festivals and culinary tours.

Thinking laterally, we might also consider policy and advocacy efforts. Those who understand the fundamental importance of the microbiome should actively advocate for policies that support microbiome research, sustainable agriculture and environmental conservation. We should emphasise the role of microbial diversity in ecosystem health, which is critical to our survival. In this regard, we must look to partnering with government agencies, non-profit organisations and industry leaders to promote microbiome-friendly practices in healthcare, agriculture and urban planning. In electronic and social media, we could develop interactive apps, websites and virtual reality experiences that allow users to explore and understand the microbiome's complex ecosystem. Along with this, we should support scientific research and technological advancements that deepen our understanding of the microbiome and its potential applications in medicine and agriculture.

Chapter 8

The current view of the microbiome

We now have a much better understanding of the five major microbiome locations, including the nasal passages, oral cavity, skin, urogenital tract and the gut. Factors such as genetics, geography, lifestyle, diet, immune system, history of infections and environment, all play crucial roles in shaping our microbiomes. One major location of the human microbiome is the gastrointestinal tract (GIT) which has the largest interface between the external environment and the body. It is one of the largest and most complex microbiomes.

Some researchers consider the GIT's microbiome as an organ in its own right[1] due to the sheer volume of microbes housed within it. The microbiome of the GIT stretches along the entire length of the gut, with approximately 100 million microbes per millilitre of saliva in the mouth alone, which reduces to thousands per millilitre in the stomach, but then increases to millions per millilitre in the ileum, the final part of the small intestine. The number of microbes reach their highest concentration in the colon where they have been measured at 10^{11} bacteria per gram of stool. In healthy individuals, microbes make up 30% to 50% of stools passed from the large intestine.

The colon's microbiome is the most diverse of all, consisting of up to 100 trillion bacteria, archaea, protists and fungi, which colonise the lumen and the intestinal walls.[2] Although much of the microbiome volume consists of bacteria, there may be as many virus particles as bacteria in the gut[3], with most being bacteriophages with bacterial hosts. Altogether, the number of microbes in the GIT microbiome exceeds the number of human cells in our body. Furthermore, the GIT microbiome contains over 22,000,000 genes[4,5], while our own human genome includes only 23,000[6]. In total, there are a thousand times more genes in the GIT microbiome than in human cells, and many are complementary to our bodily processes. This bilateral relationship relies on a complex network of molecular communication, which is poorly understood.

Bacteria are classified in a hierarchical system, like plants and animals. Here is a simplified breakdown:

1. Domain: The highest level (e.g. Bacteria).

2. Phylum: Bacteria grouped by major differenes (e.g. Bacteroidetes).

3. Class: The phyla are in turn divided into classes.

4. Order: The classes divide into orders.

5. Family: The orders divide into families (e.g. Bacteroidaceae).

6. Genus: Families divide into genera (e.g. Bacteroides).

7. Species: The most specific level (e.g., *Bacteroides fragilis*).

For example, the hierarchy for *Bacteroides fragilis* is:
- **Domain**: Bacteria
- **Phylum**: Bacteroidetes
- **Class**: Bacteroidia
- **Order**: Bacteroidales
- **Family**: Bacteroidaceae
- **Genus**: Bacteroides
- **Species**: *Bacteroides fragilis*

Identifying each microbe within the gastrointestinal tract (GIT) microbiome has been an arduous task. Most of the microbes in the GIT are harmless or symbiotic. The GIT microbiome consists of eight major bacterial phyla, typically with a combination of *Bacteroidetes* and *Firmicutes* amounting to 90% of the total. Smaller numbers of other genera of bacteria, for example, *Actinobacteria, Proteobacteria, Fusobacteria,* and *Verrucomicrobia,* are also present. The picture becomes even more complex when counting the distinct genera of each bacterium, likely encompassing thousands of different species and strains.

The majority of the *Firmicutes* are represented by various genera within the *Clostridium* group, while *Bacteroidetes* are predominantly found in the *Bacteroides* and *Prevotella* genera.[3] Actinomycetes are mostly composed of species from the *Bifidobacterium* genus, and *Verrucomicrobia* are primarily represented by the single genus *Akkermansia*. This complexity is overwhelming and hard to comprehend, and it continues to grow each day, as scientists learn more about the contents of the GIT microbiome. Despite these advances, unfortunately, our understanding of the specific roles and contributions of each species to human health and disease remains limited.

Chapter 9

How gut bacteria evolved with the human body

The microbiome has co-opted and evolved within our bodies over many thousands of years, despite the centuries of scientific ignorance regarding its place in our health. Comparisons between the genomic data of the gut microbes of humans, chimpanzees and gorillas show that our microbiomes share microbial ancestry with those animals, just as our DNA shares ancestry. Studies conducted on apes across various regions revealed an unbroken path of transmission from mother to baby spanning hundreds of generations[7]. This remarkable continuity is not a coincidence, but serves as a clue to a profound and intricate relationship.

One theory explaining the presence of the microbiome from the outset, suggests that it originally evolved to aid in the digestion of food. This theory argues that we needed bacteria to metabolise undigested food, release key metabolites, nutrients and essential vitamins that the host can then absorb. This symbiotic collaboration enabled mammals to consume a wide variety of previously undigestible foods and allowed them to survive in environments where other competing species, lacking these necessary microbiomes, would perish. By housing trillions of bacteria in our gut, humans outsourced the digestion process. In return, the microbes also thrived on the perfect temperature, anaerobic condition, moisture and nutrient-rich flow of 'chyme' (undigested food) that passed their way. This ideal symbiotic relationship continued for millions of years of evolution, that is, until the development of antibiotics disrupted this crucial balance.

To find out what role these microbiomes had in the body, researchers conducted experiments on mice and observed what would happen when all their microbiomes were eliminated. These experimental mice, sterilised of bacteria from birth, were then compared to normal mice with natural microbiomes. The results showed that sterilised mice with no microbiomes consumed 30% more calories in their diet than those with gut microbiomes. The sterilised mice developed haemorrhages and severe vitamin deficiencies[8]. Similar results were found in human studies; our gut microbes liberate about 10% more energy than would otherwise be absorbed in our diet; up to half of our daily Vitamin K is produced by gut bacteria[9]. In researching what would happen when broad-spectrum antibiotics were used in humans, human volunteers who had their microbiomes intentionally depleted also began to develop deficiencies in the coagulating protein prothrombin over several weeks[10]. These results almost mimicked the same haemorrhages that were seen in the lab mice.

Apart from boosting calorie absorption, gut bacteria are also responsible for producing numerous unique vitamins that humans cannot synthesise. For instance, gut bacteria make a significant portion of the class B vitamins we need. It is estimated that 86% of our recommended daily allowance of vitamin B6, 37% of our B9, 31% of our B12 and 27% of our B3 are synthesised by these microorganisms[11]. Our knowledge of vitamins B and K synergism is just the tip of the iceberg. Other crucial vitamins that humans obtain from external sources, such as thiamine, folate, biotin, riboflavin and pantothenic acid, are all synthesised by gut bacteria, but we have no precise information on how much is absorbed by the body.

Corollary evidence of this close relationship with our gut bacteria is provided by the existence of specialised proteins that only interact with bacteria-produced metabolites. Unlike a human enzyme, which absorbs a vitamin in its natural form, many of the enzymes on the epithelial gut surface only absorb the vitamin that is derived from and modified by bacteria.[12] This suggests we have a much more complex and dependent relationship with our gut bacteria than we once thought. Conversely, there are numerous gut microbiome metabolites which can result in harmful effects on the body, which are still in the process of being discovered. Stool-derived sclerosing cholangitis, a disease that leads to inflammation in the colon, is directly due to metabolites produced by pathogenic bacteria. This and other recent discoveries underscore the crucial role that the gut microbiome plays in our overall health and well-being.

This largely beneficial relationship between bacteria and our gut evolved to the extent that it even became interconnected with the immune system. The immune system evolved to counteract bacterial infections; however, having extensively co-evolved with gut bacteria, the immune system now had a new role – selectively cultivating friendly bacteria and eliminating pathogenic ones. Soon, complex protein interactions co-evolved on both sides of this relationship. The immune system developed protein receptors that identified helpful bacteria and left them alone, and was able to recognise and attack bacteria that were commonly pathogens, or which became too aggressive. Good bacteria stepped up this approach and developed cell-signalling messages to safeguard themselves and enlist the help of gastrointestinal immune cells[13]. So, the microbiome was not only running our digestive system: over time, it also became intricately connected to our immune system.

When researchers housed mice without gut bacteria for extended periods, these mice began to develop severe immune deficiencies that worsened over time. Mice lacking natural microbiomes experienced significant deterioration in their intestinal immune systems, including the loss of their natural intestinal mucous layer, impaired antibody production and reduced function of their intestinal lymph nodes[14.] While the symptoms in humans are not as severe, the significant increase in the incidence of gastrointestinal and autoimmune diseases, which has occurred alongside our modern use of antibiotics, tends to confirm the close interrelation between the microbiome and our immune system.

The gastro-intestinal tract houses the largest microbiome, but other microbe niches exist in almost every part of the human body. Microbes colonise our skin, nose, mucosal surfaces, respiratory tract and urogenital areas. As scientific studies in this area increase, even sites that have previously been considered sterile, such as the liver[15], blood[16] and brain[17] have been found to possess their own microbiomes. As our understanding of the intricate relationships between microbiomes and various body sites continues to expand, it becomes evident that the profound impact of these microbial communities extends far beyond the gut, reshaping our comprehension of human health and promoting new avenues of research.

Chapter 10

A microbiome theory of disease

Given that we share a close relationship with our microbiome, it follows that disruptions to it that seem harmless can sometimes lead to catastrophic health consequences. The loss of microbial diversity and stability in the microbiome has been termed 'dysbiosis'. Dysbiosis has been defined as opportunistic pathogenic bacteria becoming dominant over native species in the microbiome. The tolerance and rejection of certain species of microbes in the lumen of the gut are tightly controlled by the resident flora: since they can be affected by antibiotics and some immunosuppressants, dysbiosis can easily disrupt this ecosystem.

The most common example of dysbiosis featuring a dominant superinfection is *Clostridiodes difficile* infection. CDI is an invasive bacterial infection that secretes toxins which damage the gut lining, eventually leading to the accumulation of a thick layer of dead cells, white blood cells and mucous called the pseudomembrane[18,19]. Moreover, CDI suppresses beneficial bacteria such as *Bacteroides* and *Firmicutes*, further fuelling dysbiosis. With approximately half a million *C.difficile* infections occurring annually in the United States, resulting in around 30,000 deaths[20], it's clear that achieving the right microbial balance is not merely a dietary consideration. For many, it is a matter of life and death.

Dysbiosis, when not related to *C.difficile*, is not always so obvious. Its presence can be occult. In the context of infections, 'occult' refers to infections that are hidden or not immediately apparent. These infections may not show obvious symptoms or may be difficult to diagnose with standard tests. Occult infections can only be determined from detailed and often expensive research techniques. In other cases, dysbiosis occurs when there is an absence of some beneficial microbes. The instigating factors that lead to dysbiosis may take days or weeks to manifest, which can make diagnosis extremely difficult. CDI is one of the most acute types of dysbiosis, which can lead to gastrointestinal symptoms and possibly septicaemia (gut perforation and even blood poisoning by bacteria), but non-acute symptoms of microbiome disruption are also an active field of research. Non-acute dysbiosis has been linked to a long list of diseases including obesity, type 2 diabetes, irritable bowel disease, colon cancer, periodontal disease, atherosclerosis, endocarditis, Parkinson's disease, autism, anxiety and depression[21]. At first, there was some resistance to the idea that bacteria in the gut can affect cells as far away as the brain and give rise to cases of autism and depression. However, many researchers consider the gut microbiome a separate human organ. Under this conceptual model, just as a thymus or pancreas can signal to and control other parts of the body, the microbiome interacts similarly with both near and distant cells.

The spectacular way in which microbes communicate with their host is encapsulated in the network known as the 'gut-brain-axis', an intricate, recently discovered neurochemical link between two physically distant organs, the gut and the brain. This is no easy task, as the brain is shielded from the blood system through layers of extracellular matrix, astrocyte brain cells and endothelial cells known collectively as the blood-brain barrier. However, in both animal and human studies, when probiotics were supplied to experimental animals or human volunteers, positive neurochemical changes were detectable.

In lab mice that were genetically and behaviourally designed to have anxiety and depressive behaviours, lactic acid bacteria supplementation improved behavioural states. Feeding mice lactic acid bacteria (found in foods like yogurt) changed their brain chemistry, specifically by reducing a calming chemical called GABA in some areas of the brain, but increasing it in another important area called the hippocampus. This change helped the mice to feel less anxious and depressed, suggesting that these bacteria might positively affect moods by altering brain signals[22]. Although it can be tempting to discount the relevance of research on animals, the most compelling studies have shown that when the gut microbes of chronically ill human patients were transplanted to animals, the animals then suffered the same symptoms as the human donors[23-26]. Bacterial species such as *Bifidobacterium* have also been shown to produce GABA directly, which has a calming effect on the brain[27], as well as *Escherichia coli,* which produces the neuroactive compounds serotonin, dopamine and noradrenaline[28]. Crucially, these experiments resulted in increased GABA (with its calming effect) which reversed both anxiety and depression symptoms in mice, leading many researchers to consider the idea that anxiety, depression and possibly other mental illness might be linked to the microbiome.

The gut-brain-axis is just one of many 'axes' that are being discovered by researchers. Connections between the microbiome and the immune system, the skin, the liver, the lungs and cardiovascular health are also being validated. In the following chapters, I will delve into how the microbiome (or its absence) can significantly influence a variety of chronic diseases. I will also explore how restoration of the microbiome has the potential to cure ailments once considered incurable.

Chapter 11

The first silver bullet: Josie and Faecal Microbiota Transplantation

Our first clinic was located at 144 Great North Road, Five Dock in Sydney, in an unassuming red brick building. It had the one benefit of being long enough for us to fit in multiple clinical rooms for our growing staff. It was in that location that I performed the first faecal microbiome transplant in 1988. Since then, it has been purchased by a radiology business and turned into an x-ray unit.

My first patient was Josie, a young woman who presented with a laundry list of recurring symptoms, including severe abdominal pain, diarrhea, cramping, nausea, fatigue, blood pressure at the lower limit of normal and other symptoms that were progressively becoming overwhelming. She was unable to gain weight, had been diagnosed with inflammatory bowel disease (IBD) and appeared seriously ill when she was first referred to the Centre for Digestive Diseases (CDD). From her medical reports and her own description, she had bowel inflammation which was likely to be contributing to these symptoms. Biopsy results from colonoscopy reports showed non-specific inflammation, yet stool culture tests could find no known infectious pathogen.

After seeing several doctors who could not diagnose her condition, she felt she was 'at the end of her rope'. She had undergone multiple colonoscopies, and several specialists had identified 'colitis' (inflammation in the colon) for which she was treated, but none of the treatments provided any significant relief. She had also undergone close to 190 pathology tests. When she contacted me, she was at breaking point. She had been told she had anorexia, and her symptoms were all from stress. Following the advice of the other doctors, she was admitted to a psychiatric ward, housed with psychotic patients and scheduled to see psychiatrists for her gastrointestinal symptoms. Her case can be described as a tale of medical mismanagement and substandard care, all of which eventually drove her to reach out to me in desperation.

I well remember Josie's panicked voice when she called me from the psychiatric ward, saying: 'Dr Borody, there's all these mad people here. All these psychotic patients here, I want to sign myself out.' In the hope that she might still find some help there, I said: 'Give them another four days. If they haven't fixed your problem then, you'll have clear reason to leave, and you can sign yourself out.' Predictably, her symptoms persisted and unfortunately, Josie's time in the psychiatric ward may have done her more harm than good.

After her release, she came to the CDD clinic with her brother to see me. At the time, I was at a loss as to what to do, but I had just read an article by Ben Eiseman published in 1958[29] and I suspected something was wrong with her gut flora. The word 'microbiome' had not yet been used, so Dr Eiseman referred to 'gut flora' instead. When I looked at her medical history again and we talked further, Josie told me she had gone overseas completely well and had developed these symptoms only after returning to Australia. We knew that, because she had acquired this illness overseas, she might have a microbiome disturbance, but it was probably an unusual foreign species that we would not be able to culture in the lab, nor to diagnose with local pathology tests. That was a problem.

In Ben Eiseman's original paper, he noted that some people who had been given antibiotics would contract a serious diarrheal disease, from which up to 75% of patients would die. At the time, it was called pseudomembranous colitis. For me, there were multiple parallels between Eiseman's paper and Josie's case: she had a type of colitis, but we could not culture the bug. Eiseman's patients had a colitis, and he too could not find the bug, as bacterium *Clostridioides difficile* and its associated diseases were not even described until 1978, long after Eiseman's work. After reading his paper, though, I felt I had a potential cure that might help with Josie's colitis.

Eiseman performed faecal transplants on four patients and successfully cured them all. One patient was a 46-year-old man who had pneumonia, for which he had been given antibiotics. He became so ill after the course of antibiotics that he had non-stop diarrhea and was in a critical state and near death. Eiseman suggested to the patient's wife that, since the chances of his survival were slim, he wanted to try and restore his gut flora, in a last-ditch attempt to save him. They had nothing to lose, so they agreed to the faecal transplant without much hope of a cure. They used a nurse's stool as the transplant material and then delivered it to the patient as a rectal enema. Miraculously, within 24 hours the patient became virtually normal and was then given an additional enema. Having been critically ill and in intensive care for four weeks, he went home a few days after this second enema. In his paper, Eiseman went on to describe three additional cases which were similar, all with resolution of the patients' gastrointestinal symptoms following faecal transplantation.

When reading this and other articles, I was able to piece together crucial, and in fact, pivotal information. When Eiseman was doing this work (1950-1957), antibiotics were only just becoming mainstream. I began to speculate whether Josie's illness was antibiotic-induced. The sequence of clinical events described by Eiseman matched the preconditions for antibiotic-induced infection presumed to be by *C.difficile,* which had become endemic in some countries. Eiseman had faced a colitis of unknown origin which matched Josie's experience – colitis originating from an unknown and unculturable infection. These similarities and our lack of other treatment options gave me license to treat Josie with this simple procedure, hoping it would resolve her seemingly incurable illness. Like Eiseman's critically ill patient, Josie had nothing to lose.

I performed the faecal transplant very soon after Josie attended the clinic. Time was of the essence, given her serious symptoms and her increasing mental anguish. We conducted tests on Josie's brother's blood and stool and decided he should become our stool donor. We did the basics: we homogenised the stool, filtered it and gave it as an enema through standard tubing. We administered it several times as an enema, just as Eiseman had done. We had no protocol or standard model, as no-one did this routinely in the United States or the UK at the time. I had heard of someone trying it in some Scandinavian countries, but Josie's treatment was the first attempt in Australia. All we had was a single article – Eiseman's story of his success with faecal transplantation and the hope that Josie's mystery illness would respond to the same treatment.

After completing this first FMT, even if it was not curative, since I was simply transplanting faecal bacteria into the colon, where it was already supposed to be, I had confidence that Josie would be OK. We routinely use soap and water to wash out the colon, so I surmised that transplanting faecal bacteria would be a comparable process. As I often told my later patients, I was putting poo where poo would normally go. The risks were low, but we were mostly concerned about the treatment failing. The FMT seemed like Josie's only option at that point, but I could never have imagined the transformative impact on her life and on my research and career. She was the first of more than 50 patients to receive a faecal transplantation over the next 12 months[30.] Her case showed us the possibilities for treating and curing infections like colitis and *C.difficile* with a relatively simple procedure. But for Josie and the transformative effects of the FMT, I would never have pursued further research into FMTs or spent so much of my time advocating for their use in treating *C.difficile* and other infections.

After the procedure, Josie was a different person. Her symptoms were entirely resolved. She became completely healthy and normal again and went back to work. She was delighted – and so relieved that she invited me to her wedding and several fancy lunches. On one occasion, Josie's secretary asked me earnestly: 'Can you give me the same medication? You've made Josie so well. I want the same medicine, so I can feel that good.' I froze momentarily, as I had told Josie never to disclose what I did. I was afraid of the ramifications of treating her with a medically unregulated treatment. Josie was true to her word and did not disclose how she had been restored to health. Of course, her secretary had no idea that we had done a faecal transplant. She was under the impression that I had prescribed some sort of tablet. After the success with Josie, though, we began systematically treating patients who had similar symptoms with FMTs, and published this work a year later[30].

Chapter 12

Recognising *Clostridium difficile* infection

From research conducted in the 1970s, I learned that transplantation of faecal matter from a donor to a recipient had already been used in several patients. However, the inability to distinguish specific causes of intestinal disorders meant that these transplant procedures for conditions other than pseudomembranous colitis were often ineffective. This clouded the overall understanding of the microbiome: doctors could see that the faecal transplants worked, but they did not know why.

The rise of *C.difficile* infections in the 1970s marked a turning point. This spore-forming species of bacteria had been identified and given a name in 1935, but it was not recognised as a major cause of antibiotic-induced diarrhea (that is, where patients would develop the disease after a course of antibiotics), until 1978. Sadly, the widespread use of antibiotics such as clindamycin, broad-spectrum penicillins and cephalosporins fuelled a global *C.difficile* epidemic, with catastrophic consequences. Despite the warning signs, the further use of antibiotics such as fluoroquinolones worsened the spread and development of even more dangerous and hypervirulent strains of *C.difficile*. Today, the scourge of *C.difficile* infections continues. It is a leading cause of healthcare-associated infections and imposes a burden of about $796 million a year in healthcare costs in the USA[31]. *C.difficile* infection (CDI) is also a significant health issue in Europe, where healthcare institutions spend around €300 million annually to combat these infections alone.

Fortunately, early believers in faecal transplantation were already using this unconventional procedure to cure a range of disorders. Eiseman in 1958 reported the use of faecal transplants in antibiotic-associated diarrhea[29]. Though the specific diagnosis of CDI may not have been given, this application of FMT sparked further indications for its use in refractory diarrhea. Trials using raw or treated suspensions of faecal matter were administered via enemas, colonoscopes and gastroscopes (to the stomach). Donor samples came from self-samples, immediate partners (i.e., husband or wife, long-term partners), and relatives. Over time, donors were vetted and screened, and a 'super donor' subgroup was created, to improve the safety and efficacy of the transplantation. The super donors were generally people who, for various reasons, had never taken antibiotics.

Sadly, it would take several more decades for the value of FMT to be accepted by the medical community. At the time of Josie's FMT, few clinicians appreciated the value of faecal transplants, and some gastroenterologists even considered FMTs 'bad science'. CDI seemed unique, as it was widely known to be antibiotic-associated, with the severity ranging from minor and self-limiting to life-threatening, dehydrating diarrhea. CDI's defining characteristic, however, was that it was not curable by specific antibiotics.

Patients who seemed to have been successfully treated with antibiotics would relapse and return several weeks later, with recurrence rates as high as 60%. This rebounding became burdensome on both the physician and the healthcare system.

To worsen the predicament, medical guidelines advised further antibiotics (e.g. metronidazole or vancomycin) for an antibiotic-associated, antibiotic-triggered diarrhea. As soon as patients ceased antibiotics, the infection would relapse, either from hidden spores in the hospital environment or residual antibiotic-resistant spores in their gastrointestinal tracts. Unwittingly, patients and doctors were only sowing the seeds for future CDI infection by using antibiotics on and off in this way. Spores of *C.difficile* that were resistant to antibiotics would remain in the gastrointestinal tract, while the antibiotics supressed the 'good' bacteria, or bacteria that could not form spores. When antibiotics were ceased and the patient was assumed to have recovered, the spores of *C.difficile* remained, to repopulate the new microbiome. Patients were doomed to reinfection and relapse. This repeating cycle highlighted the urgent need for an effective alternative treatment.

Support for microbiome transplantations finally started to build as the epidemic of CDI added pressure to the search for alternative treatments. As early as 1984, Schwan[32] and colleagues used enemas of stool to treat a patient who had relapsed several times with CDI. This treatment cured this patient of relapses[32], but in other patients, similar enemas would not be as effective. Perhaps, if the enema only supplied microbes into the end of the large intestines and rectum, it was limited to restoring the microflora at the end of the large intestines.

Fortunately, oral probiotic studies in the late 1980s, using single species of yeast *Saccharomyces boulardii* and/or *Lactobacillus GG,* appeared to have some effect[33] on CDI and opened the door for further FMT use. When colonoscopy-aided methods to coat the entire large intestine with donor infusions demonstrated higher cure rates[34], the secret was out. Then, it was hard to refute the curative effects of FMT. By 2003, larger cohort groups would show that long-term remission rates could be as high as 90%, for what was once a life-threatening and persistently stubborn, chronic disease[35]. After decades of consistent scientific literature and several systematic reviews showing the robust effect of FMTs in maintaining long-term clinical remissions[32], there are few remaining doubters regarding the effectiveness of faecal microbiota transplantation in treating CDI.

Chapter 13

Ensuring safety of FMT for wider *C. difficile* treatment

With treatment success now established in CDI, further developments in the field shifted towards ways of standardising both the product used and the procedure. This would allow faecal transplants to become more accessible to the public, rather than being relegated to an experimental procedure. Ironically, the effectiveness of FMTs lay in the complexity and diversity of the bacterial ecosystem within each sample, but this virtue failed the traditional requirement of healthcare regulators, that the medicinal product be pure and the same as others in the same batch. The attempts to make faecal transplants compliant with regulations remains an ongoing challenge.

The development of faecal transplantation safety has not been without its hurdles. Rigorous donor screenings have mitigated transmission of diseases from donor to recipient, but a few instances have underscored the need for caution. Notably, there have been three reported cases of lethal complications that were directly related to FMT. The first reported death was in a patient with a complex history of comorbidities (the occurrence in a person of two diseases at the same time), including an enteral feeding tube, advanced cancer and a history of CDI relapse. This patient passed away from toxic megacolon, a complication of severe colon infection and septic shock, 48 hours after FMT[36]. While it was not clear if *C.difficile* relapse was responsible, or if there was insufficient donor screening, the event highlighted the need for extreme care whenever FMT is administered.

Another lethal case of septic shock occurred in 2019 when a drug-resistant *E.coli* species was transferred to an FMT recipient from a carrier donor[37]. The death could not be completely attributed to this *E.coli* strain, as the patient again had severe co-morbidities and major immunocompromisation. Meanwhile, twenty other subjects who received the same transplant had normal outcomes[37], but again, it suggested some contraindications for those with severely compromised immune systems.

In the third lethal report, improper procedures used in an oral FMT also led to the recipient passing away. Despite the many benefits of oral FMT, if it is oversupplied into the stomach, it has the negative risk of accidental inhalation (aspiration) into the lungs upon vomiting. This rare event occurs when the transplant fluid is implanted in the duodenum or stomach instead of the colon, and if the patient reflexively rejects the transplant or if it is overfilled. In this reported case, the FMT material inadvertently entered the lungs, causing severe pneumonia-like complications and death[38]. Though millions of FMT procedures have been performed, these three deaths are important reminders to stay vigilant in any medical procedure. However, the lessons learned from these unfortunate events have improved the safety of FMT dramatically and have made adverse events now extremely rare.

One of the modern mechanisms that ensures the safety of FMT today is the development of comprehensive exclusion criteria for faecal donors. This extensive list was established to ensure that no transmissible pathogen or disease would be transferred from the donor to the recipient. In its modern form, FMT donor criteria have now become so stringent that most of the population would fail the requirements. Hence, the term 'super donor' was coined for the small percentage of those who comply and have an effective stool.

These modern requirements contrast with the old convention of using the recipient's spouse or relative. More recent approaches have centred on institutional biobanks that service a large geographical area and specialise in donor screening, testing and the shipping of transplant-ready products. Donations in their modern form are collected from a small list of donors who are regularly tested, interviewed and follow a strict dietary, travel and antibiotic intake regime. The samples taken are tested for an extensive list of pathogens. These improvements have reduced delays in the access to transplants and have allowed many physicians, particularly in the USA, to circumvent the requirement for onerous regulatory approvals for every single transplant procedure.

The medical delivery of microbiota transplants has also become safer over time, while enormous variations in different styles of endoscopy have been attempted. Almost all transplant techniques have consistently shown high success rates (over 90%) regardless of the delivery technique. Whether faecal infusions are delivered via a colonoscope, enema, or naso-jejunal tubing, the efficacy rates are largely similar. In more recent developments, the evolution of faecal transplants into twelve orally ingested capsules (e.g. the Seres product) has avoided the need for anaesthesia and the operating room altogether. This approach, combined with safe and reliable biobanks, could extend the public availability of faecal microbiota transplantations in the future.

Overall, the case for faecal transplantation in CDI has been highly serendipitous. If not for the overwhelming success in *C. difficile* patients, the appreciation of the microbiome may have been delayed for several more decades. The fortuitous success of initial experiments with enemas in the 1950s and 1960s, although somewhat less effective, led to further attempts, using the colonoscope to deliver the transplant material higher up the large intestine, which was even more successful. Continued research in the treatment of *C. difficile* infection is far from over, but the stunning and consistent results from FMT have left very few doubters remaining.

My personal experience with FMT for CDI has shown that it is safe and effective as a first-line therapy[39]. The conventional practice of pre-treating patients with vancomycin, as mandated in the United States, may inadvertently harm the microbiome and constitutes an unnecessary aspect of CDI therapy. In a subsequent example, we will delve into the case of Coralie Muddell, who had experienced vancomycin treatment failure, persistent diarrhea and even incontinence. Initially opposed to undergoing an FMT, she eventually consented to the procedure, which ultimately proved highly effective in curing her condition.

Chapter 14

The case against microbes

An anecdote that once circulated among medical professionals goes like this: During a break from his practice, the father, from a family of doctors, had his recently trained son fill in for him as a locum. When the father returned, the son remarked 'Do you remember Mr. Phillips?' 'Of course,' replied the father. The son continued excitedly 'You've been treating his duodenal ulcer for years, right? Well, I managed to cure it!' The father paused, a faint smile on his lips as he looked away. Then he turned back to his son and asked, 'Why would you do that? Mr. Phillips practically put you through medical school!'

This joke made the rounds among gastroenterologists in the nineties because it had become abundantly clear that stomach ulcers could now be permanently cured with a regime of antibiotics. Not only were millions of lives saved around the world, with A$10 billion saved over 17 years in Australia alone[40], but the healthcare system also changed for the better. Gut surgeons in the seventies and eighties had once been drowning in endless bookings for ulcer surgery. When I was able to eradicate *Helicobacter*, the bacteria causing ulcers, the infection and incidence rates dropped so dramatically that many ulcer-oriented centres could not cope with the change. Even large, multi-storeyed centres like The Centre for Ulcer Research and Education (CURE) in the United States closed within a few short years.

These new discoveries damaged a lot of traditionally held beliefs that ulcers were caused by stress and were an incurable condition. Schwarz in 1910 underlined the role of acid in the disease with his dictum 'no acid, no ulcer' and this teaching persisted for almost a century[41]. This was in spite of the discovery of *Helicobacter*-like bacteria by Polish Professor W. Jaworski in 1896 at the Cracow Jagiellonian University[42], and initial success with multi-pronged antibiotic treatments[43]. Although in retrospect it seems obvious that *Helicobacter* was the cause, this was far from apparent at the time. There was a long-standing idea that the stomach was sterile due to its high acidity. This was supported by microbiologists' inability to grow bacteria from stomach biopsies. Additionally, antacids such as magnesium and aluminium hydroxide provided immediate symptomatic relief of ulcers, pointing to acid as the cause, and acid-reducing treatments became a profitable mainstay for treatment, which contradicted the theory that bacteria were to blame.

When H2 agonists (e.g. cimetidine) were developed in 1966, it was another step in the wrong direction. H2 agonists specifically blocked the production of acid in the stomach and provided very effective symptomatic relief. This invention by Sir James Black led to a Nobel Prize and rose in popularity with the medical community as 'the first effective drug for peptic ulcers'. As a result, even when spiral-shaped (*Helicobacter*) bacteria could be clearly seen by pathologists when slides were stained appropriately, their presence was disregarded, due to the patients' symptomatic relief. With so many patients permanently reliant on daily antacids, profits soared for drug companies and incentives to find a permanent cure for stomach ulcers were strongly opposed.

When I came back from my training at the Mayo Clinic in Rochester in 1983, I began to have suspicions regarding the treatment for peptic ulcers. At the time, we had a PhD student, Stuart Hazell, from the University of New South Wales, looking very carefully at *Helicobacter* in gastric mucosa with an electron microscope, the highest resolution microscopy technique available at the time. We were able to take high resolution photographs of *Helicobacter* from stomach biopsies and found it in two different forms – inside human cells (intracellular) and outside cells (extracellular). This was a critical discovery, because I knew that infections with an intracellular lifecycle were difficult or impossible to treat with just one antibiotic, and any antacid treatment for this bacterial problem would only provide symptomatic relief.

Both Mycobacterium tuberculosis (TB), and Mycobacterium leprae, the causes of tuberculosis and leprosy, spend much of their lifecycle within host cells. I had treated both diseases in the

Solomon Islands with two, three or even four antibiotics. To cure chronic *Helicobacter* infections, I knew that a multi-drug regime was necessary and that single drug regimens would fail. This was seen as a crazy idea at a time when most physicians were using acid tablets to treat ulcers, rather than antibiotics or multiple drug therapies. The key word here is treat, not cure. The ulcers would recur, the symptomatic relief provided by acid tablets would fade and they would be back to square one.

When dealing with intracellular infections like those from *Helicobacter*, single antimicrobial agents were not just ineffective, but a catastrophe. The history of treating TB is the best illustration of this. In the 1950s, the antibiotic isoniazid was given to people with TB, which helped many patients, but quickly led to drug-resistant TB strains and complete treatment failure for anyone unfortunate enough to be infected with a resistant strain. From practical experience, we learned that patients with TB (which we later found to be an intracellular pathogen) requires a regime of three or more antibiotics. I knew this first-hand because I was in the unique position of having spent a year in the Solomon Islands, inadvertently learning how to treat TB. I was the only doctor on this 160km island, home to more than 50,000 people at the time, and many on Malaita had TB. I treated everybody, which meant hundreds of cases, whereas most experienced doctors would not see one case back in Australia.

One of the more frustrating parts of this story was that some of the people I had started on antibiotics called Streptomycin and Isoniazid would abandon their course of treatment. Months later, I would be treating newly-infected children from the village of the runaway patient. But I would be faced with a more difficult TB strain, which was resistant to the original antibiotics I had prescribed. I then had to use up to seven different antibiotics to clear the infection completely. it was this practice that eventually persuaded me and led to the creation of triple therapy for peptic ulcers.

The bacterium responsible for leprosy behaved similarly. It belonged in the same genus Mycobacterium as TB and lived intracellularly, within its host's cells. On Malaita, we had 135 lepers living in a leper colony, whom I treated with Dapsone, Isoniazid, Rifampicin and Clofazimine. Leprosy was a completely curable disease, but it required a consistent, long-term treatment over six to twelve months. Again, multiple antibiotics were required, to eradicate the bacteria at different stages of its lifecycle. This was more difficult in Malaita because patients would sometimes stop taking their antibiotics or would not have access to a doctor for follow-up care. Unfortunately, I would see drug-resistant strains of leprosy also develop among those who had not completed their treatment.

What the medical community had not appreciated about *Helicobacter pylori* – like TB and leprosy – was that it required a combination regime of three or more antibiotics for a longer dosing period. Single agent antibiotic regimes that lasted several days, which were designed for extracellular, fast-growing bacteria, simply did not eradicate the infection. Much of the bacteria remained sheltered within the host cells until the environment became more favourable, at which point it re-emerged to wreak havoc on the patient's gastrointestinal system. Initial trials that failed using antibiotics treatments fuelled ongoing speculation that peptic ulcers were not caused by *Helicobacter*, when actually, the observations simply showed insufficient dosing, an inadequate secondary antibiotic, or insufficient treatment term. These reflections seem obvious, now that we know how to treat peptic ulcers and have conclusively demonstrated their link to *Helicobacter*. At the time, though, most physicians were severely misguided in the belief that they were caused by stress and acid.

Chapter 15

Paving the way forward

Two Australian researchers, Dr Robin Warren, a pathologist who rediscovered *Helicobacter* and Dr Barry Marshall, whom Warren took on as a research fellow, had been arguing the case that ulcers and much of their sequelae were due to *Helicobacter*. Both had worked with patients suffering from ulcers – Marshall clinically and Warren histologically. They began campaigning for the need to research beyond the outdated idea that stress and acid was the cause of stomach ulcers. However, both financial profit and the misguided convictions that antacid drugs like Zantac and Tagamet were the final solution meant there was no real incentive to find a cure. Most patients with ulcers did not need surgery and did not die, but still lived with severe discomfort.

In an interview, Dr Marshall recalled the desperation he felt at seeing patients nearly dead from bleeding ulcers, or those who had had their stomachs removed as a last-ditch attempt to save them[44]. He referenced the difficulty in the United States where doctors did not have access to the same antibiotics as in Australia, so surgery was a primary therapy before antibiotic therapy. This left many people, Barry says, 'disfigured gastric-wise' and with a dysfunctional gastrointestinal system for the rest of their lives[45]. He tried to convince others that bacteria were responsible for gastritis, but these concerns fell on deaf ears.

Like my own experience with doubtful colleagues when I proposed triple therapy for treating peptic ulcers in 1984[40], Barry's claims were dismissed, as were papers he wrote in the US on *Helicobacter*. Prominent gastroenterologists at the time simply rejected Barry's manuscripts for publication. Without published papers to validate his theories, Barry's ideas about *Helicobacter* were pushed aside.

As the saying goes, innovative ideas typically traverse three phases: disbelief, resistance (which coincided with Barry's departure for the USA), and acceptance, as if they had been common knowledge all along.

Barry went to great lengths to prove his point, ultimately consuming a beaker of cultured *Helicobacter*. Five days later, he began to have bad breath and violent vomiting attacks, waking up and having to run to the bathroom and vomit clear fluid. He had developed acute *Helicobacter* gastritis, and a second endoscopy confirmed that his stomach was overrun with the bacteria. Finally, the presence of rampant infection in his stomach had proved his theory that acute gastritis was caused by *Helicobacter*. Because he had proved it in such a spectacular fashion, people began to take notice. But he did not develop an ulcer.

Barry's gastritis went away on its own, as it does for many people. However, another researcher by the name of Arthur Morris also swallowed a concentrated culture of *Helicobacter* in New Zealand and stayed infected, chronically. Morris, though comparatively unknown, was a more accurate representative case study of the patients we encountered in our clinics. Morris, in an effort to rid himself of the infection, undertook several courses of antibiotics, one after another, and was seen by several doctors who were unable to eliminate his infection. He was seriously ill for months, without being able to resolve or eradicate the H. pylori that riddled his stomach. Finally, Morris used an antibiotic regimen from our clinic, and I successfully eradicated *Helicobacter* from his stomach.

I continued to develop a combination therapy against *Helicobacter* at my clinic in Five Dock. The combination therapies grew from dual to triple and even quad therapies. I eventually settled on a Triple Therapy comprising bismuth subcitrate, metronidazole, and tetracycline. The term 'Triple Therapy' originated from our discovery at the Centre for Digestive Diseases and our invention was eventually marketed by Procter and Gamble as Helidac.

One of the major adopters of our work came through Dr Wink De Boer from the Amsterdam Medical Centre. We were undertaking the same research and thus partnered with the Canadian company, Axcan Pharma. This connection put us in touch with Patrick McLean and

Leon Gosselin who spent much of their career marketing numerous medications, including our triple antibiotic therapy which we called Pylera – our cure for peptic ulcers.

At the time, though, doubt was still widespread. At an event for gastroenterologists, many declared we should not claim to 'cure' these ulcers, as they believed this was overstating things. I discussed this idea with my anaesthetist wife Sue at the time, who had been working closely with me for many years. We questioned ourselves and our claims: should we stop saying we were curing people of ulcers? Should we temper our claims, to fall in line with the criticism we were receiving? The people who vehemently opposed and expressed their doubts were also our colleagues and were respected in their fields. It was difficult to disregard their criticisms of triple therapy, especially given the ubiquity of antacids. In the end, we realised we were right, but it had not been an easy journey. These ideas of 'curing' ulcers created division with my colleagues, just as my later work on FMTs was debated and dismissed by so many.

Ultimately, I put a sign up behind me in my office of a quote from the German philosopher Arthur Schopenhauer. He reminds us that 'All truth passes through three stages. First, it is ridiculed. Second, it is violently opposed. Third, it is accepted as being self-evident.' A fourth stage, 'praise goes to the non-participants' was later added by Professor Wendy Hoy of the University of Queensland. This was precisely the process for people accepting the curative effect of our ulcer treatment, and I hoped it would one day be the case for microbiome research and FMTs, as well as for our therapy on Crohn's Disease, where we are on the cusp of a cure.

We were lucky with triple therapy, because we had had the unusual good fortune of being able to break through the set beliefs and reach Schopenhauer's third stage with a condition which was very common, affected millions of people every year and was easy to treat. We possessed the knowledge of a simple therapy that was able to eradicate *Helicobacter,* and we knew that once it was gone, it was truly, completely gone. Even while surrounded by doubt, we knew we had found something that would help people worldwide.

The cured patients were a testament to the effectiveness of the treatment. Before this, clinics were inundated with operations like highly selective vagotomy, an invasive procedure that permanently severed the major nerve branches connecting to the stomach. The change was dramatic. At one stage when I was looking for a job in the USA, I was interviewed by the famous researcher, Prof. Morton Grossman of the Centre for Ulcer Research and Education (CURE). He initially had difficulty accepting the concept that an infection can cause an ulcer, but later accepted my research. Several years after triple therapy was developed, the CDD changed its focus to other diseases, because we had cured ulcer disease by removing the stomach infection, *Helicobacter*. We reached that moment in curing ulcers but we are still working towards similar outcomes in numerous other infection-driven conditions.

In later years, we improved our formula to develop Pylera, an enhanced triple therapy with added Proton Pump Inhibitors, omeprazole. It went through several clinical trials and with the help of our Canadian collaborators, Patrick McLean and Leon Gosselin, we were able to take Pylera to market, world-wide. Over the next ten years, I was busy campaigning and promoting the therapy at medical conferences around the world, trying to communicate to as many people as I could how important this new therapy would be. To this day, we are continuing to improve on the formula with a product called Talicia, which comprises a single capsule of Rifabutin, Pantoprazole and Amoxycillin.

About ten years after Barry Marshall proved the link between *Helicobacter* and chronic gastritis, it was the evidence from our large cohort of Triple Therapy cures that overwhelmingly pointed to *Helicobacter* as the cause of chronic peptic ulcers. With both Barry's evidence implicating gastritis and my evidence linking *Helicobacter* to ulcers, we had established *Helicobacter* as the primary origin of the disease. Barry Marshall did not use, nor did he publish on Triple Therapy[45] but together, this finding altered many people's historical beliefs about ulcers arising from stress and acid and their subsequent treatment with antacids. Today, the idea that peptic ulcers are caused by *Helicobacter* is as clear as day. Once the infection was eradicated, the ulcers never returned. The naturally slow growth of *Helicobacter*, the acquired immunity against the bacterium and *Helicobacter*'s low infectiousness meant that once a patient was cured, they were rarely reinfected.

The recognition of this cure among the medical community was not a smooth journey. Like the doubt and opposition Barry had faced when researching *Helicobacter*, many of my well-established colleagues derided the idea of Triple Therapy as a treatment for peptic ulcers - they were still using acid suppressants like Tagamet and were loudly opposed to my therapy. A change in treatment for ulcers would mean shifting their entire idea of what caused ulcers and no longer prescribing antacids to cure them. Ironically, the resistance was strongest from gastroenterologists. General practitioners were more ready to accept the new theory, simply because the change in their patients was undeniable. General practitioners would constantly send patients to me because they could see how well this new treatment worked, and how few patients' ulcers returned. The ten years I spent campaigning to medical professionals for Triple Therapy was like building a wall, brick by brick, but I knew it was the way forward, because the cured patients were the ultimate proof.

Through a historical lens, it was Walery Jaworski who first discovered *Helicobacter*, Robin Warren who rediscovered it, Barry Marshall who proved gastritis is caused by *Helicobacter*, and our research centre that proved ulcers were caused by *Helicobacter* and provided the cure – in the form of Triple Therapies. Robin and Barry ultimately received the recognition they deserved, in the form of the 2005 Nobel Prize in Physiology or Medicine 'for their discovery of the bacterium *Helicobacter pylori* and its role in gastritis and peptic ulcer disease'.

Chapter 16

Differences between *Helicobacter* and *C. difficile*

The contrast between the treatment of *Helicobacter* and *C.difficile* infections could not have been more different. *Helicobacter* was treated with high doses of sterilising antibiotics. *C.difficile* was treated by introducing billions of faecal microbes. *Helicobacter* infection required the eradication of all microbes from the stomach. *C.difficile* was caused when a patient took too many antibiotics. The irony of the two conditions was not lost on me. It highlighted how much more we still had to learn about the mystery of the microbiome.

If there was any similarity between these two conditions, *Helicobacter* and *C.difficile*, it would certainly have been that both could kill the patient. When both bacterial species grew out of control, either in the stomach or the lower intestine, the infections could turn lethal. But the story was not that simple. An unresolved, enigmatic characteristic of *Helicobacter* was its presence in over 50% of the world's population[46], yet 80-90% of those infected had no ulcer and very minor or no clinical symptoms[47]. Barry Marshall was a case in point. He experienced the (self-inflicted) symptoms of acute infection from *Helicobacter* – vomiting, localised pain and localised inflammation, but over several days his immune system quickly cleared his infection and he was back to normal.

Arthur Morris, the unsung hero who also ingested a beaker of *Helicobacter*, could not fully eradicate his *Helicobacter* despite the use of single regime antibiotics, a plethora of doctors and specialists, and no known immunodeficiencies. Much of the general population at the time harboured asymptomatic *Helicobacter* infections over many years. Like Arthur's chronic infection, it would eventually lead to ulcers, chronic inflammatory lesions and discomfort. In a small percentage of cases, these lesions morphed into carcinomas, a cancer that forms in the tissue that lines the organs of the body. The polarity in outcomes between two seemingly similar people, Barry and Arthur, who both drank a beaker of *Helicobacter*, led some researchers to believe for a time there were protective probiotic strains of *Helicobacter* as well as pathogenic strains. Perhaps only those who had the pathogenic strains of *Helicobacter* were getting the ulcers? If in fact we had been living with and evolving with *Helicobacter* as we had with the rest of our microbiome, could it be feasible to wonder if not all *Helicobacter* bacteria behaved the same way, and that our immune system even tolerated it as a symbiote?

The strongest proponents of this idea suggested that some subspecies of *Helicobacter* played a beneficial role in the stomach, perhaps normalising the acid-reducing reflux and preventing autoimmune conditions such as asthma or inflammatory bowel disease through immunoregulation[48]. This is the ability of the body first to identify and then to eliminate organisms that are potentially harmful and to maintain equilibrium and stability within the body. These insights came after the comparison of data showing inversely growing incidence rates of autoimmune diseases, just as *Helicobacter* was being eradicated and incidence rates declined. The direct link between the elimination of *Helicobacter* and the rise of autoimmunity has remained a theory without strong evidence. Considering the uncertainty over the benefits of *Helicobacter* and the risk of harbouring a future stomach cancer, most clinicians eventually favoured *Helicobacter*'s elimination. This is in total contrast to the behaviour of the bacteria in the human gut, the microbiome. In the gut microbiome there are indeed beneficial bacteria as well as pathogens.

The differences in the effect of *Helicobacter* and *Cloistridium difficile* on their host may have arisen from their ecological niches in the gut, rather than their specific traits. While it was beneficial for both *Helicobacter* and *C.difficile* for their host to survive, the lower intestine had a dense and overcrowded microbiome, while the stomach was mostly harsh, acidic and sterile. This anatomical difference stemmed from the stomach being the gatekeeper for the rest of the digestive system. The functional role of submerging newly ingested food in strong stomach acid has the effect of sterilising and killing most of the bacteria before they pass into the rest of the digestive system.

This process protects the host from infectious diseases and eliminates rival microbes, so that the intestinal microbiome is not faced with any bacterial challengers. Based on current literature, while it appears that the lower intestine has developed a sophisticated symbiosis between the host and the microbiome, the stomach does not seem to have developed an equivalent system. Some species of stomach bacteria other than *Helicobacter* have been identified in the genera of *Streptococcus, Lactobacillus*[49]. However, even here, no specific functional role has been identified for these species, and they appear to be a residue species carried over from microbes in the saliva.

The recent identification of the species *Mycobacterium abscessus* in the stomach further affirms that there does not appear to be a positive role for these bacteria in the stomach[50]. When the native bacterial species of the stomach were assessed, *Mycobacterium abscessus* appeared to be associated with stomach ulcers in 96 out of 129 patients. *M.abscessus* also possesses the ability to colonise human cells intracellularly, a trait it has in common with *Helicobacter*. This characteristic enabled both bacteria to escape immune detection and persist chronically.

Any bacteria that inhabit the stomach maintain a fine balance between survival and disintegration. The stomach is filled, not only with gastric acid, which can denature bacterial proteins, but with aggressive digestive enzymes like pepsin, which can cleave bacterial proteins with rapid efficiency. Antibiotics in the stomach make an already harsh and unforgiving landscape an even harder place for bacteria to live and thrive.

The life of *C.difficile*, on the other hand, appears markedly different. Whilst *M.abscessus* and *Helicobacter* are commonly found in the stomach environment, *C.difficile* only appears to gain a foothold when other intestinal microbes are suppressed. In a healthy, functional microbiome, *C.difficile* exists in low to undetectable amounts, and other probiotic species in the genus Clostridioides and *Clostridium* have beneficial roles in the microbiome. Yet, when the healthy microbiome is perturbed and supressed by antibiotics, *C.difficile* expands like an opportunistic weed and establishes itself unopposed.

Key to *C.difficile*'s ability to re-establish itself, even in the presence of antibiotics, is its ability to produce a hibernating spore form of itself. Bacterial spores are metabolically dormant versions of themselves with a tough surface coating, making them intrinsically resistant to external stresses and to antibiotics. *C.difficile*, when encountering environmental stresses such as nutrient starvation, can switch cellular reproduction to the formation of spores rather than metabolically active, live forms of *C.difficile*. From the perspective of other bacteria living in the lower intestines, the introduction of antibiotics by the host is a major calamity. Spore formation therefore is an essential mechanism to ensure the continued existence for many bacteria, not only for *C.difficile*. Once bacteria are in spore form, their impermeable cell capsule is resistant to antibiotics, and the immune system may stay dormant and viable for years, whether in the gut, on hospital surfaces or in the environment[51].

In the conventional treatment of *C.difficile* infection (CDI), once antibiotics have cleared living vegetative forms of *C.difficile*, symptoms of pain and diarrhea also subsequently dissipate, but this gives a false sense of security. Even though all metabolically active *C.difficile* have been eradicated, it is rare for all sporulated (spore) forms of *C.difficile* to be eliminated. These dormant *C.difficile* spores, being metabolically inactive, give off no immune response and appear harmless, but when antibiotics are discontinued, these dormant spores germinate to vegetative forms, gain dominance in the gut and again cause severe life-threatening symptoms.

A better image of what happens in patients with recurrent CDI is the analogy of a forest ravaged by fire. When a forest fire tears through a region, it destroys most living organisms, but not all. A small minority of seeds may be sheltered underground or encapsulated in heat-resistant casings. Days after the fire, these protected seeds begin to sprout; several weeks later, the seeds and plants that once lay dormant and acquiescent on the forest floor begin to repopulate and overrun the barren landscape.

The domination of the landscape by the fire-resistant species is an intermediary period which may last years or decades. The previous biodiversity, once consisting of tall tree canopies, ferns, fungi, insects and animals, can take several decades to redevelop fully. The re-emergence of the mature, ecologically diverse forest relies on the long-term absence of further fires, or at least a period of many years to allow new plants to re-establish themselves. We can imagine what occurs when forest fires become very frequent. Fire-resistant species have more opportunities to spread over the environment after each subsequent fire. The fire-resistant seeds get produced in higher densities. As the higher frequency of fires multiplies, their population grows exponentially. Other species without this fire-resistant ability that once lived in the forest are given less opportunities to survive and repopulate the landscape.

This analogy is useful when thinking about CDI, because the fire is like the use of antibiotics. The fire-resistant species are the *C.difficile* spores, hiding in the hope of future germination. Once a complex microbiome is eradicated by antibiotics use, *C.difficile* spores remain to re-cultivate the landscape when antibiotics are discontinued. Epidemiological evidence supports this analogy, with each recurrence of CDI shown to increase after each subsequent use of antibiotics. 15-30% of patients treated with antibiotics for CDI will get a relapse of CDI. Those that have a second relapse have a 40% chance of recurrence, those who have a third relapse will have a 65% chance of recurrence[52]. Each round of antibiotics strengthens the bacteria's hold. While antibiotics may work in the short-term, like the forest fire laying waste to the trees, they set the foundations for *C.difficile* to dominate the gut microbiome in the long-term, which is why we must look to other solutions.

The realisation that long-held beliefs are wrong always prompts reassessment and valuable lessons for the future.

The traditional belief that catching a bacterial or viral infection is a matter of bad luck may be incorrect. Bombarding our bodies with antibiotics and washing ourselves incessantly may have worked in the past, but we now recognise this approach has reached its limits.

Our current understanding, based on the latest scientific findings, supports the idea that bacteria, like the organisms in the forest, each have their own ecological niche and ways of surviving. To prevent overgrowth and infection by harmful ones, we need to harness the power of good bacteria in our microbiome, to ensure that pathogenic ones cannot regenerate or take hold.

The cause of rampant overpopulation of a single toxic bacterial species is unlikely to be the result of an unlucky single encounter. It is more probable that several factors are supporting the pathogen's growth. This explains why some people may have low levels of *Helicobacter* living in their stomach and never encounter symptoms such as peptic ulcers for an entire lifetime. It also explains why low levels of *C.difficile* can also be present in the microbiome of everyday people and not lead to adverse symptoms.

Letting our microbiome run completely wild, or the inverse, obliterating it with antibiotics, are both catastrophic extremes. An unaltered microbiome can cultivate the wrong species, leading to gastrointestinal complications. Equally, bombarding the microbiome with antibiotics can lead to *C.difficile* infection. Like a careful and patient forest caretaker, a more skilful approach is to cultivate and adjust our microbiome carefully, pruning some species when necessary and giving more delicate native species time to flourish.

Chapter 17

Crossing the great divide

There was no single event that led to my confidence in microbiome transplants. It grew gradually after our success with the first patient, Josie. Her miraculous recovery changed everything and set me on this path. However, a large part of our progress after Josie was the result of reaching out to supporters in Europe and the US who were interested in our work on *Helicobacter*, a part of the gastric microbiome. So, in the late 1980s, most of my time was spent presenting at various conferences in Europe.

I had just finished presenting my lecture in Berlin in early November 1989 when I heard that the 'Iron Curtain' Wall which had divided Berlin was being dismantled. I joined the crowds walking under the Brandenburg Gate. It was incredible to witness the removal of this monumental barrier. It felt surreal to be standing there while Berlin was in turmoil. When the Berlin Wall fell, the Brandenburg Gate became a symbol of German unity. As I passed under the Gate, I kicked aside empty beer cans and champagne bottles strewn across the path, glass crunching underfoot. The nearby houses were converted into public radio stations protected by thick glass walls. As the sky faded into a velvety blue sunset, Russian troops crossed into West Berlin, bringing with them items for sale – tanks, army hats, medals and AK47s. Children perched on top of the Wall, chipping away at it to sell the pieces in plastic bags. I bought some of these Wall fragments sold by the students. Everyone wanted to feel part of the moment and share a piece of history.

Getting back to my hotel from the Brandenburg Gate was tricky, as there were thousands of people crowding the park in front of the Gate. I took a Trabant taxi, which was a cheap East German copy of a Fiat, and it turned out that the driver was also from East Berlin. He had entered West Berlin to start driving people around, except he had no idea where to go because he had never been to West Berlin before. After an unplanned tour of the city, we finally arrived at my hotel.

Despite the very foreign surroundings, the language and the differences in our work, the researchers who had invited me to speak eventually became some of my closest supporters. Many of them were intensely interested in the *Helicobacter* field at the time, so when the whole story came out, Australian researchers attracted a bit of attention. Though our medical experiences were different, we had a common interest in *Helicobacter*. I had many long conversations with the pathologists there and our collaborations eventually led to the novel discovery of *Helicobacter heilmannii*. This was an infection transmitted from dogs to humans, which led to peptic ulcers, just like *Helicobacter pylori*. It was first named in Germany, but we had seen the original specimens in Australia because we were endoscoping such large numbers of patients.

Without meeting these German researchers, we might not have identified *heilmannii* for years. Comparing our different work and medical practice across continents showed us how important it was to share our knowledge. It enabled both groups to expand our understanding of the gastric microbiome. Even though our case studies and patients were all different, as were the healthcare settings we were working in, this conference and others showed how intercontinental collaboration could work. These partnerships would be the cornerstone of our work in years to come.

My friend and colleague, Professor Robert Clancy was a researcher and clinician who had supported me for many years. We first met years before we studied *Helicobacter*. About twenty years ago, his PhD student, Jacqueline Turton cultured and identified *Mycobacterium avium paratuberculosis* (abbreviated as MAP) in patients with Crohn's Disease. This was an unpopular hypothesis at the time, but one I had long been advocating, as I watched Crohn's patients improve so markedly on Anti-Mycobacterial Antibiotic Therapy (AMAT). After seeing his student's results, Clancy became a convert and ended up supervising my PhD thesis on triple therapy for peptic ulcers. We would work late into the night, finding time for research while presenting at conferences and trying to maintain our relationships with collaborators. The work never stopped.

One of my most vivid memories was Professor Clancy's conference, held on a Russian spy ship in the Antarctic. He borrowed my laptop in the morning to give lectures and presentations and I worked on my thesis late into the night. I completed my thesis and forged a lasting professional relationship with one of the most enlightened historians, physicians and researchers I have met. This friendship has lasted for decades, right up to the present day.

Chapter 18

MS reversed in mice and men

My collaboration with Professor Clancy ignited my fascination with autoimmune diseases. At a time when medicine was achieving significant breakthroughs in eliminating infectious diseases worldwide, a new trend emerged: there was a significant rise in conditions marked by persistent and chronic inflammation without external pathogens. These conditions fell under the umbrella term of 'autoimmune diseases', as they were believed to originate from the immune system's misguided attack on the body's own cells.

In 2011, a study in the prestigious journal *Nature* demonstrated that the gut microbiota were essential in triggering autoimmune diseases. In a well-known mouse model of Multiple Sclerosis (MS), they showed that mice which should have developed MS never developed the disease when they were housed completely free of all germs and kept in totally sterile conditions. Suddenly, when these mice were introduced to normal healthy microbiota, they developed autoimmune diseases. The scientists then cross-checked and confirmed that the diseased mice had the same functional immune system as the conventional mice. They concluded, therefore, that the sole cause must have been gut microflora[53]. The results from autoimmunity studies in mice were soon reproduced in other models of autoimmune disease. Significant discoveries in diseases such as systemic lupus erythematosus (SLE – the most common type of lupus) followed. For example, it was shown that faecal transplants from mice with lupus symptoms could transfer the same bodily symptoms to recipient mice. Not only this, but genetic analysis showed that inflammation genes were upregulated in the recipient, which worsened their lupus symptoms[54].

Given the growing evidence that gut microbiota were essential to autoimmunity and treating autoimmune conditions, investigations began focusing on potential methods for therapeutic intervention. Mice mimicking MS were treated successfully with faecal transplantations from healthy mice. Clinical symptoms of the disease reduced, brain blood vessel integrity was preserved, and researchers saw reductions in the damage to brain tissue such as the axons and myelin. This was effectively the healing and reversal of MS[55]. Similar findings were replicated in mouse studies involving incurable autoimmune diseases like ulcerative colitis[56] and atopic dermatitis[57]. It is, however, worth noting that these results have not yet been replicated in humans, although numerous clinical trials are currently under way.

By this time, anecdotal evidence of the link between autoimmunity and the microbiome was already gathering. Having seen at first hand the benefits in my own patients with other co-morbidities, I documented the first three cases of patients in my care with a diagnosis of MS and what appeared to be simultaneous improvements after they received FMTs[58].

My first case involved a 30-year-old man who presented with constipation, a history of MS and a history of unsuccessful attempts to treat his conditions. His symptoms included severe leg weakness and the requirement for a wheelchair and a urinary catheter. To treat his constipation, I used five FMT infusions, which resulted in the complete resolution of the constipation. Over several weeks and months, his MS symptoms also progressively improved. He then regained his ability to walk and no longer required a catheter. Over a decade, he returned to normal function and started a transport company, becoming an avid motorbike rider in the process. While being able to walk again after an MS relapse is not uncommon, the permanent long-term disappearance of MS is extremely rare, yet this patient and two others who I will describe were without a relapse for up to 16 years.

In the second case, I saw a 29-year-old wheelchair-bound man with 'atypical multiple sclerosis' and severe, chronic constipation. He had numbness and tingling in his hands and as well as leg muscle weakness, which rendered him unable to walk. As in the first case, the patient received ten days of FMT infusions, which successfully resolved his constipation. Soon after, he also noted progressive improvement in neurological symptoms. Over time, after resolution of numbness and tingling in his hands and feet, he regained the ability to walk. For the next three years, the patient maintained normal motor, urinary, and gastrointestinal function and remained essentially symptom-free.

In the third case, an 80-year-old woman was diagnosed with MS and presented with severe chronic constipation, pain and cramping in her large intestines. She also had severe muscular weakness, resulting in difficulty walking. She received five faecal transplants, which rapidly improved her constipation symptoms, and she reported increased energy levels. At eight months, she showed complete resolution of all bowel symptoms and all neurological symptoms related to MS and she could regularly walk long distances unassisted. At follow up, a further two years after the FMT, the patient continued to be asymptomatic without relapse.

Even though we have anecdotal evidence like the cases above, the momentum for investigations and research into autoimmune conditions is limited. Small case studies have verified similar effects, including a study in Calgary, Canada, where a patient with secondary progressive multiple sclerosis (SPMS) achieved disease stability for over 10 years following a single faecal transplantation. This patient, despite having seven relapses over three years prior to the treatment, stabilised in all measures of disability after the single FMT and all functional scores for symptoms remained relatively stable over the ten following years[59]. Functional improvements were also documented in a single subject in Chicago, USA, who enrolled in a longitudinal study for one year. Over this period, the subject regained their ability to walk, increased their walking speed and improved gait and co-ordination in their walking. These smaller studies provided support for a larger, more robust human clinical trial to assess the validity of microbiota transplantations, but more information is still needed. These anecdotal successes need to be replicated in larger-scale studies and ongoing research.

A handful of other cases in autoimmune disease are also worth mentioning. In 2011, I published the results of a patient with spontaneous resolution of the classic autoimmune condition, idiopathic thrombocytopenic purpura (ITP)[60]. This condition arises from the immune system destroying blood-clotting platelets in the blood, leading to low levels of platelets. Before transplantation, the patient's platelet levels were beneath the lower limit of normal, reaching as low a level as 30,000 platelets per microlitre. In the months following, the patient experienced a rise in her platelet count (average 127,000 platelets/uL) which then normalised to the normal range (190,000/uL) in 2004, where they remained, even ten years later.

This kind of long-term follow up is key to our autoimmune research, because autoimmune diseases are prone to remission and relapse. In a separate case in Beijing, China, a patient with rheumatoid arthritis of five years appeared to be successfully treated with FMT. Over a period of 78 days, autoimmune antibodies significantly diminished, as did their symptoms and joint discomfort. Throughout the follow up, they were also able to reduce immunosuppressive medication significantly[61]. These cases speak not only to the immediate efficacy of microbiota transplantations, but also significant long-term improvements in the patients' experience. They too suggest a need for further, larger-scale studies to investigate why multiple FMT treatments could be a solution.

The current study of autoimmunity is somewhat in limbo. Many critics have attributed patients' 'mysterious' remission to immunosuppressive therapy or, more simply, to the unpredictable nature of relapse and remissions. Nevertheless, recovery in our treated patients after FMTs has been increasingly frequent, and we feel optimistic that larger clinical trials will provide further encouraging results.

On the other hand, progress in clinical trials has met with several setbacks. In late 2019, a large, randomised phase II clinical study aiming to treat relapsing forms of MS was terminated due to the primary investigator passing away. The study had unfortunately not recruited adequate numbers of participants, and the incomplete published data was inconsistent and inconclusive[62], so it did not present significant new findings.

A more recent, moderately sized phase II study looking into psoriatic arthritis also failed to show demonstrable results against control treatments[63], without a clear explanation for the disparity. Like the unpredictable nature of the conditions we study, the road through clinical trials has been rocky and erratic. Yet, we will only learn more about FMTs and the microbiome in autoimmune conditions through such further trials. More work on the effectiveness of multiple FMT infusions and long-term follow-up of patients should be undertaken. In the meantime, much of the microbiome's role in autoimmunity is still shrouded in mystery.

Chapter 19

FMT's effects on Parkinson's and Alzheimer's

My first interest in the connection between neurodegenerative diseases and the gut microbiome began with a patient I treated in 2009. This 73-year-old patient had been diagnosed with Parkinson's Disease (PD), with a four-year history of severe constipation. At the time, I was aware that symptoms of constipation could precede the onset of Parkinson's Disease by up to ten years. After treating the patient's constipation with a combination of antibiotics and anti-inflammatory medication, a dramatic improvement in Parkinson's symptoms also occurred. These included the loss of tremors, loss of arm rigidity and micrographia (small and cramped writing). Other classic symptoms of Parkinson's were also reversed.

Though the theories of a relationship between the gut microbiome and neurodegeneration were still in their infancy, I proposed the idea that bacterial or even fungal toxins in the gut may have been the causative factor, and that antibiotics therapy could clear these toxins and even cure the patient. Immediately after antibiotics were administered, followed by FMT in two patients with PD, constipation symptoms resolved, as well as other symptoms of PD. I personally took one of these patients back to his neurologist and asked for him to be examined for symptoms of PD. The neurologist stated bluntly that he would not diagnose PD in this patient if he had presented like this, indicating that all PD symptoms had gone. This patient, who lives in a country town south of Sydney, remained well during follow-up over several years.

It was some time before animal models confirmed a similar story. While there were several theories surrounding the cause of

Parkinson's Disease itself, one theory proposed that it was caused by the aggregation of a 'wild type', malformed – the protein α-synuclein. Magnetic Resonance Imaging (MRI) of patients showed higher levels of these insoluble protein aggregates in the brain. Our suspicions about the connection between the α-synuclein and Parkinson's grew when mice were genetically modified to overexpress αSyn and developed motor deficits and activation of immune cells in their brains. When these mice were treated with antibiotics to eliminate their gut bacteria, their symptoms disappeared[26]; when they were given faecal transplants from human Parkinson's patients, their disease symptoms got worse. This pointed to PD faecal flora as the cause of PD.

Further sequencing-based research confirmed the connection and the pathways involved. By sequencing the RNA (Ribonucleic acid, the molecule that exists in the majority of living things and viruses) of the gut bacteria from these sick mice, some bacteria stood out, such as *Firmicutes* and *Clostridiales*, which appeared at much lower levels, while *Proteobacteria*, *Turicibacteriales* and *Enterobacteriales* were higher[65]. Unusually, the levels of bacteria-fermented metabolites called short-chain fatty acids were also increased. When FMTs were performed on these mice, the Parkinson's-like physical impairments recovered, dopamine and serotonin receptors in the brain returned to normal[66], short-chain fatty acids decreased, and neuronal immune cells became less activated. These studies were also replicated in other types of PD mouse models[67], where repairing their gut flora helped to bring about drastic improvements in their symptoms. Interestingly, patients after total vagotomy are less likely to develop PD, indicating that the neurotransmission pathway has been partially blocked to αSyn travel.

The theory that gut microbiota could permit the transfer of neurotoxins to the brain via axonal transport was plausible enough to implicate another devastating neurodegenerative condition – Alzheimer's Disease. In a similar style of research, mice were genetically modified to express a different protein, the amyloid precursor protein, which is known to turn into the amyloid-β protein. Amyloid-β protein was like the αSyn of Parkinson's and was found to be concentrated and tangled within the brains of severely affected Alzheimer's patients. When these mice grew to adulthood, they displayed premature signs of dementia and other classic signs of Alzheimer's Disease. When their gut RNA microbiota were sequenced, the researchers also found large rifts in the types and amounts of bacteria present[68]. When these genetically modified mice were raised in germ-free environments, such that their gut had no bacteria, their brains had drastically lower levels of the proteins that acted as precursors to Alzheimer's. When the faecal transplants from the sick mice were carried out in those without a gut microbiome, the brains of the recipient mice increased in amyloid-β protein. When the faecal transplants from healthy wild mice were transferred to mice without a gut microbiome, there was less amyloid-β protein than usual.

The question then turned to whether cognitive deficits could be reversed in these diseased Alzheimer's mice. After faecal transplantation from healthy mice into these diseased mice, there were improvements in their learning and memory time when put through maze tests. Using MRIs, scientists were also able to demonstrate reduced amyloid-β deposition in the brain as a result of FMT. Other proteins suspected of causing neurocognitive deficits were also decreased[69] as the mice's learning and memory time improved. These studies were replicated by other groups, independently showing reduced cognitive deficits and paving the way for further research. While we are still years away from any kind of cure for Alzheimer's, understanding these links between the gut microbiome and neurodegenerative conditions are promising first steps.

Now that we understand that symptoms such as constipation can precede neurodegenerative changes, it comes as no surprise that major microbial dysbiosis - a bacterial imbalance from an occult infection in the gut microbiome - is likely. When deeper analyses on the bacterial species of the gut were performed, many changes in the microbial metabolites in the blood were associated with changes in the brain[70]. Case reports of Parkinson's symptoms spontaneously resolving, similar to my observations in 2009, were reported by other researchers in 2019[71]. In a study in Guangzhou, China, a 71-year-old patient with PD experienced a tremor in his legs which disappeared following faecal microbiota transplantation. However, after two months, the tremor returned to one, but not both, of his legs. This was another indication that FMTs could prove useful in treating Parkinson's symptoms, but it could not be claimed to be curative. However, for patients suffering from Parkinson's, even some small relief in these symptoms – particularly motor control – is a huge step forward. With the theoretical grounding for a potential therapy in PD, three clinical trials have evaluated the use of FMT for PD. In 2020 at Nanjing University, fifteen PD patients underwent FMTs. Five of these received transplantation through nasogastric tube but showed no significant changes to their PD symptoms. Conversely, of the ten patients who received transplantation via colonoscopy, all significantly improved in their levels of sleep quality, depression, anxiety, non-motor symptoms and daily living activities[72]. These improvements were also maintained for several months.

Then in 2021, a smaller study was run with six PD patients; three showed improvements in non-motor symptoms over 1-3 months, but overall PD symptoms only improved negligibly[73]. Oddly, another notable clinical trial in 2021 used FMT in eleven Parkinson patients, but this study recorded only microbial changes in the gut and constipation, without any assessment of neurological or cognitive changes[74]. While changes in the gut and constipation are promising, the lack of data on neurological changes severely limits the value of this study.

With so few completed clinical trials, the results are still inconclusive. There is clearly some potential in using FMT to decrease symptoms, but how FMTs affect symptoms long-term, not months but years down the line, is unknown. In the meantime, any avenue towards reducing patient discomfort and improving quality of life is certainly worth pursuing, especially with the wide-ranging benefits we have seen from FMTs in other conditions.

FMTs for the treatment of Alzheimer's Disease are even less conclusive. As with the Parkinson's research, there are some reported case studies showing success. In 2020, my collaborator measured improvements in an Alzheimer's patient's cognition, rising from a score of 20 on the standardised cognition tests, to a score of 26 two months after FMT. The patient then scored 29 on cognition tests, six months after the transplant[75]. A 90-year-old patient in South Korea also improved cognitive function by standardised testing following an FMT. This patient improved from a severe cognitive impairment of 15 to a score of 20 by the end of the study[76]. Despite the promise of these two studies, wider clinical trials with larger patient numbers have not yet been completed.

Our own research group also trialled an approach with combination antibiotics in a small pilot trial. Six Alzheimer's patients were given antibiotics and we found four out of six patients had improvements in their memory and cognition[77]. Overall, however, progress in clinical trials has been slow. This may reflect competing drug strategies being the primary focus of large drug companies, or a lingering medical attitude that continues to disregard the connection between the gut and the brain.

Chapter 20

The challenge of Autism

About 15 years ago, I had an extremely mischievous young patient named David, whose parents, Susie and David, came to see me because their son was struggling with chronic constipation. They told me he had also been diagnosed with Autism. At the time, I had a small office at 144 Great North Road, Five Dock in Sydney, with my books and journals filling the shelves along the walls. Almost as soon as he arrived, David started to tear all the books and manuscripts off the shelves, expressing his discomfort and displeasure at being in yet another doctor's office. Neither of his parents could rein him in, and a wrestling match between David, his father and me ensued, to prevent my office being completely destroyed. Eventually, David's father and I managed to gain the upper hand and pinned him to the floor.

Although Autism is considered a regressive developmental disorder of the mind, most autistic children also experience a suite of gastrointestinal problems. David was one such case and his chronic constipation was causing serious problems for both him and his family. After examining David and considering his symptoms, I treated him with oral vancomycin, an unabsorbable antibiotic which stimulates bowel emptying. When he returned, six weeks later, his constipation had all but gone, his bowel motions were near normal, and he was well behaved and receptive to his mother's instructions. The constipation had clearly been closely associated with gut discomfort, but also his cognitive dysfunction was exacerbating his anxious and repetitive behaviour. The changes in his mood, conduct and behaviour were remarkable.

The rationale for administering vancomycin to David was its limited gastrointestinal absorption. When ingested orally, it typically traverses the digestive tract and is excreted in the faeces. When taken in tablet form orally, its primary impact is on the contents of the gut, so here was a way to modify the microbiome without affecting the rest of the body. This meant it was an ideal drug to resolve David's gastrointestinal symptoms, and downstream, to influence his Autism.

Vancomycin as a treatment strategy would also be discovered by the paediatric gastroenterologist, Richard Sandler from Rush University Medical Centre in Chicago, and infectious disease specialist, Dr Sydney Finegold. Dr Sandler noted cognitive improvement after using vancomycin[78], while Dr Finegold described abnormal *Clostridia* in the gut microbiome in autistic children, which suggested systemic neurotoxins were being produced by species of pathogenic organisms in the gut. These causative bacteria could be suppressed or even eliminated by vancomycin, leading to the resolution of some of the symptoms of Autism and some of the associated gastrointestinal issues.

Dr Finegold had conducted some large-scale studies, comparing the bacterial microbiome of autistic children with non-autistic children of the same age. Much of Dr Finegold's work confirmed what we were suggesting: there were abnormally abundant species of *Clostridia,* and another type of bacteria called *Desulfovibrios* present in autistic children. *Clostridia* in particular was associated with gastrointestinal (GI) symptoms and repetitive behaviours in autistic children[79]. *Desulfovibrios* also produced toxins, and we believed we could help to relieve some of these children's symptoms, using various different methods, including antibiotics. In David's case, the vancomycin targeted these bacteria in his gut; it helped to resolve his GI symptoms and fixed other behavioural issues.

After our success with David, we started to work more closely with a microbiologist in Drummoyne in Sydney and develop our own anaerobic laboratory. We were realising that while we could keep 'bad bacteria' at bay with vancomycin, we ultimately wanted to add good bacteria as well, so we could limit the long-term use of vancomycin and promote sustainable gut health. The vancomycin had worked with David, but we needed to find a longer-term solution for people with chronic GI issues.

Leila, the microbiologist, had a building that housed CO_2 tanks, bacterial incubators and -80° freezers. She used old-school traditional forms of bacterial culture to grow small containers of non-pathogenic *Clostridia* for children to take home. When the small containers were opened, the kids wrinkled their noses and told us they smelled like 'farts'. After several weeks of drinking these probiotics in yoghurt, both their bowels and their brains improved. We had a speech therapist measure their vocabulary and speech patterns: in some cases, their speech increased from 23 words to 100 words in only a few weeks. David's vocabulary reached more than 600 words, enabling him to have fuller conversations with his parents.

After we had successfully treated twenty kids, the word was out, and we had an influx of demand. However, the regulations surrounding the administration and treatment of children had become significantly more challenging. Suddenly, we needed elevated management requests and a mounting set of approvals to treat kids, which put an end to our promising mini-trial in Australia. Many parents would still call, attempting to book their children in for FMTs. They had heard that FMTs could help resolve their children's symptoms and wanted anything they could find to make their child feel better or make their own lives easier. But we had to turn them away. On the other hand, my American collaborators were still keen and had access to funding, so several large trials were undertaken at Arizona University. With my colleagues Alex Khoruts and James Adams, we were eventually able to prove the effectiveness of FMTs and probiotics in treating GI symptoms in autistic children. A lot of time and money has been spent studying the effects of gut microbiota on Autism in the intervening years, but this work all started from my initial meeting with David and observing how profoundly the FMT affected him.

Long before I met David, the earliest clues to the link between Autism and the gut microbiome came from epidemiological data. We know that some seven out of eleven autistic children have gastro intestinal issues, but initially it was unknown if this was due to the selective eating behaviour of the children or other external factors. Improvements to DNA sequencing gave us a clearer picture of the differences between the gut microbiome of autistic and non-autistic children.

Unsurprisingly, when the gut microbiomes of autistic children were analysed, they differed significantly. The gut microbiota of autistic children contained higher amounts of pathological species such as *Clostridia*, *Desulfovibrios*, *Bacteroides* and *Ruminococcus*. Beneficial, synergistic bacteria such as *Prevotella* and *Firmicutes* were present, but in significantly lower quantities, and non-autistic children possessed higher levels of *Bifidobacterium*[80]. At the time, how these bacteria affected the brains of autistic children was still unknown, but it was clear that the microbiomes were significantly different, and we needed to learn more about them.

One theory proposed that the gut might produce pathogenic microbial metabolites, which could negatively affect the brain, exacerbating the symptoms of Autism. Bacterial metabolites such as p-Cresol had already been found to be more abundant in autistic patients than non-autistic ones. In a study where mice were exposed to p-Cresol for four weeks, they began to experience classic signs of Autism including reduced social interactions, repetitive behaviour, anxiety, hyperactivity and cognitive deficits. These mice also exhibited decreased activity of their central dopamine neurons.

To obviate all other possible causes, the faecal microbiota of healthy mice were transferred to the sick mice – whereupon the social interactions, anxiety levels and dopamine levels in the unhealthy mice returned to normal[81]. It is highly improbable that Autism is caused by one single metabolite, but the fact that the microbiota of autistic individuals is so very different from non-autistic people makes it likely that gut dysfunction does indeed have a significant effect on the brain. In the mouse study, many of the symptoms of Autism were at least a little improved after a faecal transplantation to introduce good bacteria into the gut.

Having established that gut bacteria could influence symptoms of Autism, researchers questioned whether we could replace or modify the gut microbiome to relieve some of these symptoms. In a model of Autism developed in rats, supplementation with *Bifidobacteria*, known to be 'good bacteria', resolved the rats' social behavioural impairments and increased levels of oxytocin in their brains[82].

Similarly, in another Autism mouse model, giving mice the probiotic *Lactobacillus reuteri* and oligofructose plant extracts improved their sociability by 30% and reduced repetitive behaviours by 50%[83]. Crucially, mice that consumed both probiotics and plant extracts also reduced intestinal permeability by up to 30%[83]. We know that many autistic children have high intestinal permeability, that is when bad bacteria (or even normal bacteria) can cause immune reactions in the colonic tissue and lead to mild colon inflammation. This can become an ongoing gastrointestinal problem but can also lead to more serious risks if the bacteria pass from the colon into the bloodstream or the rest of the body. Medical literature is now saturated with numerous animal studies like the ones described above. However, the true test for whether we can generate real therapies with long-term benefits for autistic children can only be determined by large clinical trials.

Due to the prevalence of gastrointestinal issues in autistic children, there are many case reports of faecal microbiota transplantations (FMTs) improving symptoms of Autism. In one case, an autistic individual, the recipient of antibiotics which may have affected their microbiome, was followed for several years. After modifications to antibiotic use, this patient reported improvements in their mental state, increased engagement in family activities and becoming calmer[84]. They were then treated with an FMT, which was consumed orally over the course of fourteen weeks. Remarkably, their Autism symptoms reduced by 4 points and empathy behaviour scores increased by 7 points compared with their old test scores, a huge improvement[85]. These results independently verified how faecal transplantation had so remarkably helped my patient, David.

In a larger clinical trial performed in China, forty autistic children were treated with FMTs. The results showed blood levels of neurotransmitters changed and the microbiome diversity shifted dramatically. The levels of a disease-associated bacterium also declined and accordingly, their Autism measures, such as mood, behaviour and emotionality, improved by 10% at a four-week check-up. The beneficial effects, however, dropped to 6% by the eighth week. By the twelfth week, Autism symptoms returned to original levels[86]. Although the study successfully treated the GI symptoms of the children, the lack of permanent change in Autism symptoms significantly challenged the theory that the microbiome was solely responsible. Despite this disheartening result, the commitment to develop a long-term solution for autism and to enhance the quality of life for these children has persisted.

Having observed that faecal transplants had only a temporary effect on Autism, we wondered if variations in the transplantation procedure and the selective use of antibiotics could be more effective. In our study in Arizona, USA, eighteen subjects underwent faecal microbiota transplants which included antibiotics, bowel cleansing and stomach acid suppressants[87]. The antibiotics and bowel cleanse were used to eliminate any unfriendly gut microbiota present, and the supplementation of acid suppressants was hypothesised to allow the newly introduced microbiota transplants to engraft themselves better in the host.

Over a two-year follow up, 66% of subjects dropped from the severe Autism diagnosis, meaning they no longer met the 'severe' criteria, and 44% of the entire group fell below the criteria for Autism altogether, meaning they were no longer classified as autistic. Bacterial sequencing of their gut microbiota showed higher microbial diversity at two years follow-up than at the eighteen weeks post-transplant, indicating a long-term improvement. These findings also suggested that studies with short follow-ups might not capture the full extent of the benefits from FMT and that supplemental medications could extend the efficacy of the treatment. Although these results were promising, we still have a long way to go with this research. Patients like David served as the starting point, offering us a glimpse into the potential of Faecal Microbiota Transplants in the future.

Chapter 21

Advancing medical knowledge – risky but rewarding

Every year since February 2005, our nurse Sharon and I would receive a long-stemmed rose, delivered to our clinic. Even though Sharon has now retired, the clinic continues to receive this annual gift. It comes with a note:

To the world you may be one person, but to this one person, you are the world.

Sincerely,   Coralie   Muddell.

Coralie's story shows how, once a wrong idea is implanted, it is hard to dislodge. Coralie was a successful pharmacy assistant, treated unsuccessfully for *C.difficile* infection by other doctors with a plethora of different treatments. Her multiple courses of vancomycin failed, and her symptoms of diarrhea returned many times. She had several consultations with me and the other doctors at the Centre for Digestive Diseases. We all told her the same thing: the only way to get rid of the infection was to repair her bowel flora with an enema of stools from a super-donor, who was special for the simple reason that they had never received antibiotics. When we described this procedure to her, she walked out of the clinic in a huff, clearly not believing any of it. Even though Coralie knew what *C.difficile* was and how serious it could become, she was not convinced by the idea of FMTs.

Several days passed and her symptoms had not abated. In the intervening period she had a minor car accident. Due to her ongoing gastrointestinal issues, she ended up soiling herself and the seat of her expensive car. Days later, she returned reluctantly to our clinic and agreed to try the procedure. We scheduled two microbiota enema infusions which, at this point, long after our first FMT patient, had standardised. Soon after the enema infusions, her symptoms disappeared. Coralie was so thankful that she could work again and travel from home to her two pharmacies, as she had before her symptoms started. She felt she had been given her life back. Every year since, she has sent Sharon and me a long-stemmed rose with the message above. She also offered her story and photos for our publications.

It can be difficult to appreciate how the quality of life changes for a person with CDI or other colon infections when the symptoms become overwhelming and uncontrollable.

Ironically, those most experienced and senior in the medical field were the hardest to convince of the efficacy of FMTs. Coralie was a pharmacist and, like many others in medicine, was strongly opposed to the idea of microbiome transplantation. However, unlike many others, Coralie had the personal distress of gastrointestinal misery and the experience of being cured. She hit rock-bottom and was desperate, yet despite having a recurrent CDI, she initially refused treatment. She was so firmly resistant to FMT that it took a personal calamity to change her mind.

This was the case with many others in the medical community, where the resistance to FMT was strongest among those experienced and knowledgeable. However, most of them did not have the personal experience that Coralie had. This opposition trickles down from researchers and organisations into everyday patient-facing practice. Even when FMTs may be able to help people with debilitating chronic conditions, it is prohibited. We have seen many cases like Coralie, who would have continued suffering indefinitely if she had not taken a chance on the new treatment. Seeing the incredible change in a patient's quality of life after successful treatment reminds us why pursuing this work is so important, and why medical research should continue to explore it.

I was in Washington at a Digestive Diseases conference when I received a call from my practice manager, Nick Shortis. He said, 'You are currently on TV, and the President of the Society of Gastroenterologists of Australia has just called you a charlatan.' The TV show was called *Charlatans* and was aired as a segment of *Good Morning Australia*. The journalist leaned in on the television monitor display controlled by the President of the Society and showed a mouse curser hovering over a photo of me in a newsprint article. They had named me and the clinic as frauds on public television.

It was not uncommon for us to get attention from different media outlets when news of faecal transplants was reported. Whenever the newsdesks requested commentary, I would respond directly. Whether it was the television news, on radio or in the newspaper, I just told people about it. In my collection of media quotes is one that says, 'if you tell the truth long enough, in the end it will find you out.' I lived by this idea and would always just tell the truth: the patients got better, and despite the external controversy, they would always be on our side.

At one stage, a long time ago, our clinic was short of patient referrals. Some doctors had to 'walk the streets' to different health centres to get patient referrals. Part of our job as specialists was to persuade general practitioners to refer patients and inform them about the use of FMTs. GPs were some of our biggest advocates, once they saw the efficacy of our treatments, unlike many researchers, as they were patient-facing. They knew the patient's diagnosis and saw the improvements after an FMT. We tried many ways to show GPs our treatments and convince them of their importance. We gave 'information dinners' to explain what we were doing and why we did it. We would book out a whole restaurant to make an occasion of it. We showed slides of our treatments and explained the science of FMT.

At this stage, the US had not caught up with our work on *C.difficile* and FMTs and there was no FDA statement on *C.difficile*. We wanted to explain our science to everyone we could, so people like the President of Gastroenterologist Society of Australia would be receptive rather than critical of the new treatment. That did not work. It did not work because we received too much media attention, which ruffled some feathers. The President of the Society set up a new rule that any gastroenterologist in the Society who wanted to speak on television or radio had to appoint the official spokesperson from the Society. The Society did not want anybody else to comment.

At that time, we were the biggest gastroenterology unit in Australia, with the most experience in triple therapy for *H pylori* and FMT. We did our own research and trained our own PhD students. There was no reason to hide. We went ahead, ploughed on and importantly the patients were on our side. Even so, medical practice would take a long time to change. Today, the FDA still requires evidence of a failed attempt at treating *C.difficile* with vancomycin before an FMT is even considered. This means two courses of antibiotics, six to ten weeks of failed treatment, more expense for the patients and pain and discomfort throughout.

It is clear that FMT should be used as early as possible, to halt the disease and limit a patient's pain. However, regulations in most countries force all physicians to follow outdated rules that have not caught up with the evidence. This is exactly why cases like Josie's are so important. If we had not treated Josie with FMT, her symptoms would have persisted and worsened, with no end in sight. Treating her was a huge risk for the clinic and my own medical practice, but it was worth it, to push our knowledge a tiny step further and to save Josie from ongoing pain.

Chapter 22

Treatments old and new

Most people have only learnt about or heard of Faecal Microbial Transplantation in the last few years. It is often forgotten that FMT as a medicinal procedure began thousands of years ago, in China. The history of antibiotics and the evolution of antimicrobials has also been forgotten in the century following the discovery of penicillin in 1928. It was an exciting, historic event, and it laid the foundation for almost all of our present day antibiotics.

Most people have heard about the discovery of the very first antibiotic, the one that changed the game. Penicillin was discovered by Dr. Alexander Fleming (1881-1955) when he returned from a summer vacation to find mould was preventing the growth of his experimental colonies of *Staphylococcus*. He concluded that this mould was acting defensively, preventing the growth of the *Staphylococcus* bacteria. He named it penicillin. It would take fourteen more years of breakthroughs in bio-fermentation to improve the yields of penicillin to the point where they could be used to treat the very first patient, but even so, it is important to remember that penicillin in its original ecological niche was produced to defend against rapidly growing bacteria.

Several more antibiotics would be identified from microbes in the natural environment in subsequent years, but not before deadly outbreaks of antibiotic-resistant infections became a serious threat. Only a few years after the first administration of penicillin, in the 1960s, deadly outbreaks of antibiotic-resistant *Staphylococcus aureus* (staph infection) plagued hospitals in the USA and the UK, exacerbated by hospital overcrowding, the ubiquitous use of penicillin and a post-war baby boom. At the height of the epidemic, more than 80% of hospital-acquired staph infections were resistant to penicillin[88]. With only one antibiotic at their disposal, doctors were helpless to treat staph infections. It was a challenge desperately needing a solution. The search was on for another antibiotic that could eradicate the penicillin-resistant strains of staph infections.

New antibacterial microbes were cultured from the soil, compost and far-flung regions of the world, in the hope of finding the antibiotic that was so badly needed. One high yield group of bacteria, the *Actinomycetes*, resembled fungi, so soil microbiologist Selman Waksman (1888-1973) theorised that this group could yield a new class of antibiotics. Given *Actinomycete's* co-existence with numerous strains of pathogenic bacteria, Selman was sure that a compound could be extracted with similar properties to penicillin. Penicillin, despite its great effect on gram-positive bacteria, was almost ineffective against another class of bacteria called gram-negative bacteria, which caused significant morbidity and mortality worldwide.

True to Selman's intuition, a systematic screening programme, subsidised by the pharmaceutical company Merck, identified *Streptomycin* from the species *Streptomyces griseus,* which would later be found to be highly effective against many gram-negative bacteria, most importantly against Tuberculosis (TB)[89]. Further antibiotics would be cultured from the *Streptomyces* species, including Chloroamphenicol, Chlorotetracycline, and then Ivermectins from *actinomycete Streptomyces avermitilis*. Such antibiotics would play a major role in eliminating urinary tract infections, pneumonia, brucellosis, the plague, typhus, severe tonsilitis, parasites and salmonella infections. This rush of new medicines looked as if it would finally stamp out most of the diseases that had plagued humanity since the dawn of civilisation.

This time has been described by many as a golden era for medicine. It began in 1928 and ended near the start of 1953, with the discovery of what many still consider one of the most effective antimicrobials: vancomycin, a poorly absorbable molecule taken orally, with which I have treated innumerable patients. However, by the middle of the 1950s, the impact of newer antibiotics contributed less to infectious disease mortality[89] every year, as the availability of antibiotics became standardised and hospitals developed multi-drug regimens that inhibited the rise of drug-resistant strains.

Vancomycin was developed by Eli Lilly from a soil bacterium found in Borneo. It possessed a remarkable ability to remain effective against staph infections (*S. aureus*) despite staph's ability to develop resistance quickly against all other antibiotics. It was also approximately twenty thousand times better than penicillin in quelling these infections. When ushered into clinical use, vancomycin quickly became one of the most successful antibiotics against penicillin and its relative, staph infection (MSRA)[90]. For many in the health field, the challenge of antibiotic resistance appeared resolved with the discovery of vancomycin. Consequently, many of the financial incentives to encourage the discovery of new antibiotics also dried up.

At the end of this golden era, these new antibacterial agents needed a name. Even though today we recognise them all as antibiotics, there was no consensus on that name at the time. In 1942, Selman Waksman proposed the term 'antibiotic' to refer to 'a compound produced by one microorganism, which is capable of killing or inhibiting another'[91]. The term came from the older French term 'antibiosis', which the Frenchman, Jean Paul Vuillemin (1861-1932) had coined in 1889 to refer to the antagonistic effects of microorganisms on each other[92]. Here, we are beginning to see how terminology from the 1940s about antibiotics intersects with our current discussions of the microbiome.

In the last one hundred years, many in the healthcare sector have come to consider antibiotics as synonymous with sterile capsules in blister packaging, but their true origins are from microbes. An antibiotic was a compound that was produced by one microorganism that inhibited another, as it was originally defined. Through the passage of time, we have lost sight of the true nature of antibiotics. They were manufactured by the chemist and the laboratory, but they belonged to the world of microbes. Although many bright minds have identified the microbe as a powerful weapon and distilled its purest form into medicines, they have also failed to appreciate the powerhouse that generated it all in the first place – the microbe itself.

The idea that all microbes were inherently dangerous was only half the story. To their unappreciated credit, microbes such as *Penicillium*,

Streptomyces and *Amycolatopsis* produced some of our best-known antibiotics, and this was just a thin slice of the microcosm. My thoughts on this crystallised when I came across a PhD student's experiment: a healthy person's stool was dissolved in nutrient agar and left to grow. Nutrient agar is a standard ingredient used in microbiology. It forms a thick jelly on which bacteria should thrive. We know that 50-80% of the dry weight of stool is composed of gut bacteria. The student expected an abundance of bacteria to grow on the agar culture plate, but after several days, nothing grew. The bacterial antibiotics had inhibited all growth.

It would be remiss not to appreciate the similarities between this PhD student's experiment and Dr Fleming's agar culture dish in 1928. Bacteria in our microbiome will be critical to the next generation of medicines. In both Dr. Fleming's and the PhD student's cases, bacterial colonies were inhibited from growing on traditional culture dishes; in Dr Fleming's case, the causative agent was mould; in this PhD experiment, it was the thousands of natural antimicrobial agents already in the stool, which were preventing the growth of microbes.

The student's experiment was a stool equivalent to Dr. Fleming's discovery of penicillin: in both cases, the growth of 'bad bacteria' was inhibited. However, in Dr. Fleming's case he won a Nobel Prize, and antibiotics became ubiquitous in western medicine. This parallel discovery related to microbes in stool was largely overlooked, even though its implications could be just as striking as Fleming's discovery of the first antibiotic.

Beneficial bacteria from the PhD experiment, such as those in the group *Bifidobacteria,* were known to be associated with a range of health benefits such as the prevention of colorectal cancer, diarrhea, colitis and irritable bowel disease, but how they work was not yet understood[93]. A closer analysis of their molecular mechanisms found that they produce antimicrobial agents such as bifidin and biflong that limit the growth of other bacteria around them[94],which is why, in the PhD experiment, nothing grew on the culture. Many bacteria in our microbiome act in this same manner and keep us healthy by producing thousands of antimicrobial compounds which act against known pathogens.

Our microbiome houses trillions of microbes, many of which produce their own anti-microbial factors. In the case of disease, the microbiome may need to be treated with antibiotics, if it cannot get rid of an infection on its own. However, in future we will probably use capsules to deliver microbiota and restore the normal gut flora. FMT has the potential to be applied to a wide range of diseases, such as irritable bowel syndrome (IBS), Crohn's disease, coeliac disease and various autoimmune disorders. Recent discoveries have shed light on the fact that the healthy microbiome has provided us with its own natural antimicrobial defences. This explains why our bodies, in return, have safeguarded this microbiome for millions of years. It is imperative that we further our understanding of this intricate relationship.

Chapter 23

Dealing with dysbiosis

Unfortunately, even though the idea that 'all bacteria are bad' has been mostly dispelled, we may have adopted yet another wrong idea: the concept of dysbiosis. Dysbiosis has been used as a microbiome-centred explanation for mysterious gastrointestinal symptoms, but the exact microbial events in dysbiosis have never been clearly defined. Some researchers have defined dysbiosis as either the sudden overgrowth of pathogenic gut bacteria, or the loss of commensal (good) bacteria, but an explanation for why this imbalance occurs is not given. The concept of bacteria being 'unbalanced' is an easy idea to understand and convey to others as an explanation for ill health. However, it may be entirely incorrect when referencing the gut microbiome[95]. Many definitions of dysbiosis suggest that it arises from any change in the composition of resident 'good' bacteria communities, compared with those in a healthy individual. In the case of Inflammatory Bowel Disease, helpful groups of bacteria (*Firmicutes* and *Bacteroides*) are suppressed[96] and the pathogenic bacteria (*Enterobacteriacea & Mycobacterium avium*) increase[97]. Comparing the diversity of bacterial species also shows that 25% less microbial diversity is found in IBD patients. This is just one example of how bacterial imbalance can cause gastrointestinal symptoms that are often generalised as 'dysbiosis'. Why this imbalance occurs is unexplained. Could it be that, as with Eiseman's patients, this imbalance is rooted in the overgrowth of an elusive pathogen, akin to the situation with *C. difficile* before its discovery in 1978?

The evidence for bacterial imbalance simply led many researchers to attribute the cause of those diseases to dysbiosis. Yet, as in the discovery of *C.difficile* infection, the abundance and disproportion of good bacteria originates from the overgrowth of *C.difficile*, and the loss of good bacteria also comes from *C.difficile* growth and its toxins. The idea of 'dysbiosis' and the perturbed gut microbiome appears the same as that seen by the original pioneer for stool transplantation, Ben Eiseman in 1957. Eiseman was unaware of the causative species *Clostridioides difficile*, which was not named until 1978. From his perspective, his patients had ruinous gut microbiomes and a clinical state almost identical to what we would now classify as 'dysbiosis'.

It seems that dysbiosis might be a lazy explanation of gastrointestinal disease when a cause is unknown. If we continue thinking that dysbiosis equals disease, it becomes easy not to investigate any further. This is also true for other conditions like autoimmune diseases. Many clinicians will say that an inflammatory process causes autoimmune disease without looking further upstream for a definitive cause. In these cases, patients are often prescribed anti-inflammatory medications, on which they become reliant, while the real problem is simply symptomatically suppressed. We need to look at the whole picture. As doctors and diagnosticians, we should ask ourselves which pathogen caused the dysbiosis or a 'disturbed' microbiome in the first place.

In the case of *C.difficile* infection, once we had identified the causative species, we no longer classified *C.difficile* as dysbiosis, because it was understood that *C.difficile* was suppressing the growth of other beneficial commensal species. In fact, it was *C.difficile* (the pathobiotic) which had become overabundant and was causing patients' gastrointestinal symptoms, often driven by the toxins it produced.

With further developments in medicine, we uncovered other forms of pathobiotic groups such as *E.Coli, Campylobacter, Salmonella* and *Staphylococcus*. These species are only a handful among a superabundance of trillions of bacteria in the gut microflora, most of which we can not yet culture in the laboratory. Among the bacteria that modern science has identified, only 30,000 have been formally named and are kept in pure cultures, yet our estimates of the number of unique species of microbes on earth is close to one trillion.

There is still much we do not know about the microbiome and many species that have not yet been cultured or named. The term 'dysbiosis', as it is currently used in research, might be a catch-all phrase for the manifestation of a microbial infection, but just like in Eiseman's cases, we have not yet identified the causative microbe. It is still not known whether dysbiosis in some cases is caused by a singular infective agent. If and when we discover this, the concept of dysbiosis will become even more irrelevant.

One reason why we have been clinging to some of these mistaken ideas for so long may have had something to do with the gut biofilm. Biofilms are semi-solid films, comprising irregular layers of mixed populations of bacteria, archaea, bacterial DNA and other microbes that adhere to living and non-living epithelial mucosal surfaces. Microbes, it turns out, love to live in biofilms. Biofilms allow microbial communities a safe harbour against varying temperatures, pH, oxygen radicals, salinity and other extremes that can easily cause their demise.

Everyone is familiar with the sticky white substances that form on our teeth after a sugary meal, which is in fact a type of dental biofilm. By adhering to the tooth surface, the microbes have easy access to the food that the host eats and a perfectly warm and moist environment. If they did not adhere to the tooth's surface, the microbes would be washed away along with the rest of the food into the stomach and eventually destroyed by stomach acid. Similarly, biofilms in the colon can embed and attach to the gut epithelium (inner lining) to resist being eliminated from the gut with the moving mass of stool.

Researchers are currently debating whether the presence of these thick diverse biofilms in the gut mucosa are beneficial or pathogenic. However, their existence does suggest why *C.difficile* infection is so hard to remove solely with antibiotics. We can deliver antibiotics to the bloodstream and within the lumen digestive space of the gut, but so far, we have rarely attempted to deliver antibiotics to the biofilm, where some key microbes take shelter. This explains why *C.difficile* can still reside in the gut despite multiple rounds of antibiotics. It also explains why, in a small minority of cases, faecal transplantation is unsuccessful, because *C.difficile* is still hiding within this thick, resistant, biofilm matrix.

The gut biofilm, however, is not just a host for pathogens. Its very existence explains another microbiome phenomenon – bacterial species returning to the host gut lumen even after long periods of antibiotic treatment. Antibiotics lead to significant drops in the microbiome, but they rarely sterilise it completely. In almost all cases, the gut microbiome recovers, occasionally with a different composition from the original. In mice model experiments, strong doses of the antibiotic streptomycin reduced bacteria in mouse stools more than 100,000-fold[98]. Yet, despite ongoing antibiotics, the anaerobic bacteria recovered to the previous levels within the second day. We can only account for this sudden reconstitution of bacterial abundance, if a buffer and refuge that is impervious to antibiotics is available for microbes in the colon– and that is most likely the biofilm.

In sequencing experiments taken directly from this biofilm layer in mice, we saw that this bacterial community retained higher species richness than in the empty lumen spaces of the intestines. Prior to antibiotic treatment, both the lumen and the biofilm layer held similar species richness, yet following antibiotic treatment, the mucus-associated biofilm lost much less bacterial diversity than the luminal communities[99]. Antibiotics also led to specific groups of bacteria, such as *Proteobacteria,* increasing in the lumen, and conversely *Clostridia,* responsible for increased CDI, in the biofilm layer. Both observations explain why *C.difficile* infection is resistant to antibiotic treatment and how it can return even after treatment, given the ideal conditions to thrive[100].

The gut biofilm is likely a mechanism that helps the host to repair the microbiome after damage. In a cross-examination study featuring 117 individuals and 782 microbiome profiles, bioinformatic mining of this dataset uncovered 21 bacterial species that exhibited robust association with bacterial diversity when recovering from antibiotic therapy[101]. These included *Bacteroides thetaiotaomicron* and *Bifidobacterium adolescentis,* which promoted microbial recovery at least 100 times faster than without their presence. In this data, there were also no apparent 'bad bugs' that thwarted recovery[102]. This information is revelatory. It also dispels the long-held, third principle in Koch's postulates, that '*The cultured microorganism should cause disease when introduced into a healthy organism.*'

Our growing understanding of the gut biofilm is beginning to suggest that the *absences* of key bacteria, as well as the presence of microbial pathogens, may promote gut disease. This also teaches us that our gut can be exposed to a pathogen and recover well. What seems important is that we store the correct 'good bugs' in our gut. Perhaps the original biofilm was intended to work to restore our original microbiome. If our microbiome falters, we can use a transplantation from a super donor. This explains why FMT has been so effective; because it is inconsequential whether we hold 'bad bugs.' We simply need enough of the 'good bugs' in our biofilm to overwhelm the bad ones, which make us ill.

With this knowledge, though, we must also realise the limitations of our own techniques, because FMT in its current form uses only stool samples or the 'shed bacteria from the biofilm'. Our modern practice of faecal transplantation takes bacteria from the super donor and reintroduces them into the lumen space of the sick patient. If the modern theory of the biofilm is correct, then more effective strategies would involve transplanting super donor biofilm species directly into or onto the patient's own biofilm[102], thus giving them the 'good bugs' they need.

Some of the answers to our most difficult and incurable diseases might be lying in plain sight. I was once raked over the coals by the medical establishment for my outlandish ideas in stool transplantation, specifically by the President of the Gastroenterological Society of Australia. The late British neurologist, John Hughlings Jackson expressed it best when he said…

It takes 50 years to get the wrong idea out of medicine and 100 years to get a right one into medicine.

No one wants to stand up and have their research shot down, and few doctors and researchers can bear rejection from major funding sources or risk their medical licences to practise being terminated. Hence, the stakes are always high for both the doctor and the patient. When I treated Josie, I risked my medical licence and my ability to get research funding, in the hope that an FMT would resolve her symptoms. Thankfully, it worked, but had it not been successful, our later discoveries might never have happened. To make progress, we must be open to new ideas, even if they seem strange at the time. The complexity and alien nature of the microbiome is such that virtually anything is possible. If we are not careful, we could completely miss discovering what really matters and how to treat it.

One can never be certain of the future, but I suspect that a Nobel Prize will come to the person who can reliably cure most of the diseases that arise from the microbiome. We are getting very close to this result in *C.difficile* treatment, with many reviews reporting over 95% of patients achieving long-term remission, but we have not been able to cure anywhere near 100% of patients with Ulcerative Colitis and Crohn's Disease. We know that there is a strong connection between the gut microbiome and Autism, as well as autoimmune diseases, Multiple Sclerosis and Parkinson's disease. In our own clinic we have seen patients with Multiple Sclerosis and Parkinson's Disease rid themselves of their wheelchairs after being successfully treated with FMT. The hard work is getting closer to that 100%, and some of those answers may lie buried in the biofilm. It always starts with a single case or a single patient, like Josie, David or Coralie. These cases become omens for the future, pointing the way forward and reminding us that if we persevere, we can change the face of disease for all our future patients.

So, what is the future of the human microbiome, in research, treatment and understanding?

Advances in research have identified microbial diversity and have continued exploring this diversity across populations and environments. This will deepen our understanding of how microbiomes influence health and disease. In addition, advances in metagenomic sequencing and bioinformatics will enable more comprehensive analyses of microbial communities, identifying novel species and functions. With medical applications through microbiome-based therapies, we will see the development of microbiome-targeted therapies, such as probiotics, prebiotics, FMT and microbial engineering, to treat various diseases and disorders.

Medical applications will also see the integration of microbiome data into personalised medicine approaches, to tailor treatments based on an individual's microbial profile and health status. To this should be added technological innovations like microbiome engineering, where advances in synthetic biology and genetic engineering make it possible to manipulate microbial communities for therapeutic or industrial purposes. Also important is the development of non-invasive diagnostic tools and biomarkers based on microbiome signatures, to predict disease risk and monitor treatment outcomes.

While there have been considerable attempts in this area and papers that indicate a connection between neurodegeneration and the microbiome, there is still a long way to go with our research. We need to know why FMT improves some patients' symptoms and not others, and how it affects the acceleration or slowing of disease. As knowledge currently stands, human studies and clinical trials in this area are significantly underpowered and under-developed. While it is clear that gut bacteria are significantly altered by neurological disease, there remains an unknown knowledge gap: why do some patients not respond to FMT? Or why do their symptoms return sooner in some conditions than in others?

A more radical theory is that Parkinson's and Alzheimer's may be a long-term consequence of gut dysbiosis, and short-term therapy might just be an intervention coming too late. Those with the most severe symptoms may have neuronal damage far too advanced to be rescued. Even so, stratification and patient selection with 'mild' cognitive impairment and recently diagnosed neurodegeneration would help to answer the question of whether microbiome treatments could be more effective.

Chapter 24

The microbiome and YOU

I promised to take you on a long journey through my life's work and we have almost arrived at the present. We have witnessed vast armies of microbes doing battle over the internal organs of real, live human beings, just like you and me. And I have shared some of the personal battles fought along the way, between medical researchers seeking to understand the inner workings of our bodies, in the hope of establishing new, effective treatments for some of the many ills that flesh is heir to. We medics can be a combative lot, but our overriding aim is to help people to feel and be better, so they can enjoy their lives untroubled by sickness.

I apologise for having inflicted so many long, unfamiliar words on you, but when we identify a new species of microbes, we name them – in Latin, of course, so that medics all over the world will use the same names. Imagine if we had to translate them all into a multitude of different languages. Like botanists, we need to use a universal language, so that we can share our knowledge, our hypotheses and our discoveries. As scientists, we regularly share our work in academic papers, so that researchers of all nations can cooperate to find the answers to our common problems. No doubt, a million minds are better than one.

The fundamental change that has happened in my lifetime is that mass communications have allowed patients to access the latest medical research. Dr Google has a lot to answer for – but it must be beneficial for medical knowledge to be more widely accessible than ever before – even if we humans have an irresistible temptation to over-simplify everything. Perhaps that compensates for scientists tending to over-complicate matters.

It is now a truth universally accepted that 'we are what we eat'. The question few people ask themselves is 'how does what we eat become us?' The answer to that absorbing question lies in the microbiome – and the purpose of this book is to help you to understand a little more about the microbial universe that exists in every one of us.

As I theorised in Chapter 9 (paragraph 2), in the course of evolution, we have effectively outsourced our digestion to the microbial communities inside us – and we have also entrusted them with maintaining our health, and even our existence, in the face of pathogenic attacks.

We can see a parallel to this on a much larger scale. In Australia, we are familiar with the concept of invasive species. In almost two and a half centuries, since the first white settlement, we have imported (usually with the best motives) many species which have gone on to occupy a more prominent environmental niche than we intended for them: rats, mice, rabbits, foxes, feral cats, camels, wild horses, cane toads and now fire ants have all accepted our invitation to call Australia home. Environmental scientists are battling to keep them under control, just as the 'good' microbiota in our microbiomes try to master the pathogens.

It is only right that we should share the emerging knowledge about our own bodies. When I first practised medicine in the Solomon Islands, my patients had no access to the internet or even to books. Nevertheless, they still sometimes knew more about their condition than I did. It is the diagnostician's job to watch and listen carefully, to reflect and seek for clues, which are often provided by the patients themselves.

These days, patients in developed countries often present at the medical centre, having self-diagnosed and studied online about what they think is their complaint. This can be a help or a hindrance to the GP, but there is no point complaining about it, because a vital part of human progress is the acquisition of more knowledge. The key question is what we do with it.

The same process is already taking place with the microbiome. People have learned that their diet has a huge impact on their internal flora, so they seek out prebiotic foods, rich in fibre, such as onions, garlic, bananas, oats, barley, apples, avocado, asparagus and seaweed, as fuel for their beneficial gut bacteria. When they believe there is a need to repair actual damage to their microbiome, they take probiotic foods, containing live micro-organisms, like yoghurt, kefir or buttermilk and other fermented products, such as kimchi, sauerkraut, miso, soy sauce and sourdough bread. It would be great if we could simply undo all the damage we have caused with antibiotics by taking a few probiotics – but I doubt if the solution is going to be that simple.

This is a very inexact science: how do you know you are taking the best supplement for your regular diet, in the ideal quantities, at the most advantageous times? It is a little like trying to hammer in a nail with a shovel: it might work, but you probably won't know if it has until it's too late. Doctors try hard to choose, not only the right medication, but the correct dosage. However, these attempts at self-medication, are certainly preferable to the alternative where people simply eat whatever they fancy, with no regard to its effect on their health, weight and wellbeing. At least people are beginning to understand that our microbiomes deserve close attention.

There is a great public appetite for knowledge about the way our bodies work and the effects on them of the exercise we take (or fail to take) and the food we eat. This little book is an attempt to share what I have learned in the course of a lifetime studying the microbiome.

I have been privileged to work on one of the frontiers of medical science. My work has been patient-focused from the first, and my interpretation of the needs of my patients has led me to try and find new solutions for their problems, even at the cost of courting controversy. Many people still have an instinctive, visceral reaction to the concept of Faecal Microbial Transplantation – but I have witnessed this treatment giving new hope and new life to patients who were at the end of their tether.

My appeal to my colleagues in the medical profession, to funding bodies, charities, governments and, first and foremost, to you, the readers of this book, is to beg for further attention to be paid to this branch of medicine. From my own experience, I believe it may hold the clues to unravelling some of the most perplexing puzzles facing medical science. I believe that presently incurable conditions, such as MS, Crohn's, Parkinson's, Alzheimer's and Autism may either originate or be exacerbated by conditions in the microbiome. There is a chance here, however slim, to relieve the suffering of millions of people, worldwide. We will not have definitive answers to these questions until costly, large-scale clinical trials are commissioned and completed.

REFERENCES

1. Baquero F. Nombela C. The microbiome as a human organ. Clin Microbiol Infect. 2012 Jul;18 Suppl 4:2–4.

2. Sender R, Fuchs S, Milo R. Revised estimates for the number of human and bacteria cells in the body (Internet). bioRxiv; 2016 (cited 2023 May 4). p. 036103. Available from: https://www.biorxiv.org/content/10.1101/036103v1

3. Reyes A, Semenkovich NP, Whiteson K, Rohwer F, Gordon JI. Going viral: next-generation sequencing applied to phage populations in the human gut. Nat Rev Microbiol. 2012 Sep;10(9):607–17.

4. Tierney BT, Yang Z, Luber JM, Beaudin M, Wibowo MC, Baek C, et al. The Landscape of Genetic Content in the Gut and Oral Human Microbiome. Cell Host Microbe. 2019 Aug 14;26(2):283-295.e8.

5. Qin J, Li R, Raes J, Arumugam M, Burgdorf KS, Manichanh C, et al. A human gut microbial gene catalogue established by metagenomic sequencing. Nature. 2010 Mar;464(7285):59–65.

6. Aebersold R, Agar JN, Amster IJ, Baker MS, Bertozzi CR, Boja ES, et al. How many human proteoforms are there? Nat Chem Biol. 2018 Mar;14(3):206–14.

7. Moeller AH, Caro-Quintero A, Mjungu D, Georgiev AV, Lonsdorf EV, Muller MN, et al. Cospeciation of gut microbiota with hominids. Science (Internet). 2016 Jul 22 (cited 2022 Jan 21); Available from: https://www.science.org/doi/abs/10.1126/science.aaf3951

8. Gustafsson BE, Daft FS, Mcdaniel EG, Smith JC, Fitzgerald RJ. Effects of vitamin K-active compounds and intestinal microorganisms in vitamin K-deficient germfree rats. J Nutr. 1962 Dec;78(4):461–8.

9. Hill MJ. Intestinal flora and endogenous vitamin synthesis. Eur J Cancer Prev. 1997 Mar;6 Suppl 1:S43-45.

10. Frick PG, Riedler G, Brögli H. Dose response and minimal daily requirement for vitamin K in man. J Appl Physiol. 1967 Sep;23(3):387–9.

11. Magnúsdóttir S, Ravcheev D, de Crécy-Lagard V, Thiele I. Systematic genome assessment of B-vitamin biosynthesis suggests co-operation among gut microbes. Frontiers in Genetics (Internet). 2015 (cited 2022 Jan 20);6. Available from: https://www.frontiersin.org/article/10.3389/fgene.2015.00148

12. Intestinal absorption of water-soluble vitamins: an update - PubMed (Internet). (cited 2022 Jan 20). Available from: https://pubmed.ncbi.nlm.nih.gov/16462170/

13. Tordesillas L, Berin MC. Mechanisms of Oral Tolerance. Clin Rev Allergy Immunol. 2018 Oct;55(2):107–17.

14. Johansson MEV, Jakobsson HE, Holmén-Larsson J, Schütte A, Ermund A, Rodríguez-Piñeiro AM, et al. Normalization of Host Intestinal Mucus Layers Requires Long-Term Microbial Colonization. Cell Host Microbe. 2015 Nov 11;18(5):582–92.

15. Leinwand JC, Paul B, Chen R, Xu F, Sierra MA, Paluru MM, et al. Intrahepatic microbes govern liver immunity by programming NKT cells. J Clin Invest. 2022 Apr 15;132(8):e151725.

16. Castillo DJ, Rifkin RF, Cowan DA, Potgieter M. The Healthy Human Blood Microbiome: Fact or Fiction? Frontiers in Cellular and Infection Microbiology (Internet). 2019 (cited 2023 May 4);9. Available from: https://www.frontiersin.org/articles/10.3389/fcimb.2019.00148

17. Link CD. Is There a Brain Microbiome? Neurosci Insights. 2021 May 27;16:26331055211018708.

18. Levy M, Kolodziejczyk AA, Thaiss CA, Elinav E. Dysbiosis and the immune system. Nat Rev Immunol. 2017 Apr;17(4):219–32.

19. Frosali S, Pagliari D, Gambassi G, Landolfi R, Pandolfi F, Cianci R. How the Intricate Interaction among Toll-Like Receptors, Microbiota, and Intestinal Immunity Can Influence Gastrointestinal Pathology. J Immunol Res. 2015;2015:489821.

20. Lessa FC, Mu Y, Bamberg WM, Beldavs ZG, Dumyati GK, Dunn JR, et al. Burden of *Clostridium difficile* infection in the United States. N Engl J Med. 2015 Feb 26;372(9):825–34.

21. Warinner C, Speller C, Collins MJ, Lewis CM. Ancient human microbiomes. J Hum Evol. 2015 Feb;0:125–36.

22. Bravo JA, Forsythe P, Chew MV, Escaravage E, Savignac HM, Dinan TG, et al. Ingestion of *Lactobacillus* strain regulates emotional behavior and central GABA receptor expression in a mouse via the vagus nerve. PNAS. 2011 Sep 20;108(38):16050–5.

23. Ge X, Zhao W, Ding C, Tian H, Xu L, Wang H, et al. Potential role of fecal microbiota from patients with slow transit constipation in the regulation of gastrointestinal motility. Sci Rep. 2017 Mar 27;7(1):441.

24. Transferring the blues: Depression-associated gut microbiota induces neurobehavioural changes in the rat - PubMed (Internet). (cited 2022 Jan 26). Available from: https://pubmed.ncbi.nlm.nih.gov/27491067/

25. Gut microbiota from multiple sclerosis patients enables spontaneous autoimmune encephalomyelitis in mice - PubMed (Internet). (cited 2022 Jan 26). Available from: https://pubmed.ncbi.nlm.nih.gov/28893994/

26. Sampson TR, Debelius JW, Thron T, Janssen S, Shastri GG, Ilhan ZE, et al. Gut Microbiota Regulate Motor Deficits and Neuroinflammation in a Model of Parkinson's Disease. Cell. 2016 Dec 1;167(6):1469-1480.e12.

27. Yunes RA, Poluektova EU, Dyachkova MS, Klimina KM, Kovtun AS, Averina OV, et al. GABA production and structure of gadB/gadC genes in *Lactobacillus* and *Bifidobacterium* strains from human microbiota. Anaerobe. 2016 Dec;42:197–204.

28. (Amine neuromediators, their precursors, and oxidation products in the culture of Escherichia coli K-12) - PubMed (Internet). (cited 2022 Jan 25). Available from: https://pubmed.ncbi.nlm.nih.gov/19845286/

29. Eiseman B, Silen W, Bascom GS, Kauvar AJ. Fecal enema as an adjunct in the treatment of pseudomembranous enterocolitis. Surgery. 1958 Nov;44(5):854–9.

30. Borody T J., George L, Andrews P, Brandl S, Noonan S, Cole P, et al. Bowel-flora alteration: a potential cure for inflammatory bowel disease and irritable bowel syndrome? Medical Journal of Australia. 1989;150(10):604–604.

31. Finn E, Andersson FL, Madin-Warburton M. Burden of *Clostridioides difficile* infection (CDI) - a systematic review of the epidemiology of primary and recurrent CDI. BMC Infectious Diseases. 2021 May 19;21(1):456.

32. Schwan A, Sjölin S, Trottestam U, Aronsson B. Relapsing *Clostridium difficile* enterocolitis cured by rectal infusion of normal faeces. Scand J Infect Dis. 1984;16(2):211–5.

33. Gorbach SL, Chang TW, Goldin B. Successful treatment of relapsing *Clostridium difficile* colitis with Lactobacillus GG. Lancet. 1987 Dec 26;2(8574):1519.

34. Persky SE, Brandt LJ. Treatment of recurrent *Clostridium difficile*-associated diarrhea by administration of donated stool directly through a colonoscope. Am J Gastroenterology. 2000 Nov;95(11):3283–5.

35. Aas J, Gessert CE, Bakken JS. Recurrent *Clostridium difficile* colitis: case series involving 18 patients treated with donor stool administered via a nasogastric tube. Clin Infect Dis. 2003 Mar 1;36(5):580–5.

36. Solari PR, Fairchild PG, Noa LJ, Wallace MR. Tempered enthusiasm for fecal transplant. Clin Infect Dis. 2014 Jul 15;59(2):319.

37. DeFilipp Z, Bloom PP, Torres Soto M, Mansour MK, Sater MRA, Huntley MH, et al. Drug-Resistant E. coli Bacteremia Transmitted by Fecal Microbiota Transplant. N Engl J Med. 2019 Nov 21;381(21):2043–50.

38. Baxter M, Ahmad T, Colville A, Sheridan R. Fatal Aspiration Pneumonia as a Complication of Fecal Microbiota Transplant. Clinical Infectious Diseases. 2015 Jul 1;61(1):136–7.

39. Roshan N, Clancy AK, Borody TJ. Faecal Microbiota Transplantation is Effective for the Initial Treatment of *Clostridium difficile* Infection: A Retrospective Clinical Review. Infect Dis Ther. 2020 Dec 1;9(4):935–42.

40. Eslick GD, Tilden D, Arora N, Torres M, Clancy RL. Clinical and economic impact of 'triple therapy' for *Helicobacter pylori* eradication on peptic ulcer disease in Australia. *Helicobacter*. 2020;25(6):e12751.

41. Fatović-Ferenčić S, Banić M. No acid, no ulcer: Dragutin (Carl) Schwarz (1868-1917), the man ahead of his time. Dig Dis. 2011;29(5):507–10.

42. Konturek JW. Discovery by Jaworski of *Helicobacter pylori* and its pathogenetic role in peptic ulcer, gastritis and gastric cancer. J Physiol Pharmacol. 2003 Dec;54 Suppl 3:23–41.

43. Rigas B, Feretis C, Papavassiliou ED. John Lykoudis: an unappreciated discoverer of the cause and treatment of peptic ulcer disease. Lancet. 1999 Nov 6;354(9190):1634–5.

44. Discover Magazine (Internet). (cited 2023 May 31). The Doctor Who Drank Infectious Broth, Gave Himself an Ulcer, and Solved a Medical Mystery. Available from: https://www.discovermagazine.com/health/the-doctor-who-drank-infectious-broth-gave-himself-an-ulcer-and-solved-a-medical-mystery

45. Professor Barry Marshall, gastroenterologist | Australian Academy of Science (Internet). (cited 2023 May 31). Available from: https://www.science.org.au/learning/general-audience/history/interviews-australian-scientists/professor-barry-marshall

46. Graham DY, Malaty HM, Evans DG, Evans DJ, Klein PD, Adam E. Epidemiology of *Helicobacter pylori* in an asymptomatic population in the United States. Effect of age, race, and socioeconomic status. Gastroenterology. 1991 Jun;100(6):1495–501.

47. Cleveland Clinic (Internet). (cited 2023 May 31). H. Pylori Infection: How Do You Get, Causes, Symptoms, Tests & Treatment. Available from: https://my.clevelandclinic.org/health/diseases/21463-h-pylori-infection

48. Owyang SY, Luther J, Kao JY. *Helicobacter pylori* : beneficial for most? Expert Review of Gastroenterology & Hepatology. 2011 Nov;5(6):649–51.

49. Koga Y, Ohtsu T, Kimura K, Asami Y. Probiotic *L. gasseri* strain (LG21) for the upper gastrointestinal tract acting through improvement of indigenous microbiota. BMJ Open Gastroenterol. 2019 Aug;6(1):e000314.

50. Chouhan D, Barani Devi T, Chattopadhyay S, Dharmaseelan S, Nair GB, Devadas K, et al. Mycobacterium abscessus infection in the stomach of patients with various gastric symptoms. PLoS Negl Trop Dis. 2019 Nov 4;13(11):e0007799.

51. Paredes-Sabja D, Shen A, Sorg JA. *Clostridium difficile* spore biology: sporulation, germination, and spore structural proteins. Trends Microbiol. 2014 Jul;22(7):406–16.

52. Song JH, Kim YS. Recurrent *Clostridium difficile* Infection: Risk Factors, Treatment, and Prevention. Gut Liver. 2019 Jan;13(1):16–24.

53. Berer K, Mues M, Koutrolos M, Rasbi ZA, Boziki M, Johner C, et al. Commensal microbiota and myelin autoantigen cooperate to trigger autoimmune demyelination. Nature. 2011 Nov;479(7374):538–41.

54. Ma Y, Xu X, Li M, Cai J, Wei Q, Niu H. Gut microbiota promote the inflammatory response in the pathogenesis of systemic lupus erythematosus. Mol Med. 2019 Aug 1;25(1):35.

55. Li K, Wei S, Hu L, Yin X, Mai Y, Jiang C, et al. Protection of Fecal Microbiota Transplantation in a Mouse Model of Multiple Sclerosis. Mediators of Inflammation. 2020 Aug 5;2020:e2058272.

56. Treatment and mechanism of fecal microbiota transplantation in mice with experimentally induced ulcerative colitis - Leichang Zhang, Xiaofei Ma, Peng Liu, Wei Ge, Lixia Hu, Zhengyun Zuo, Huirong Xiao, Wu Liao, 2021 (Internet). (cited 2022 Mar 1). Available from: https://journals.sagepub.com/doi/abs/10.1177/15353702211006044

57. Kim JH, Kim K, Kim W. Gut microbiota restoration through fecal microbiota transplantation: a new atopic dermatitis therapy. Exp Mol Med. 2021 May;53(5):907–16.

58. Borody T, Leis S, Campbell J, Torres M, Nowak A. Fecal Microbiota Transplantation (FMT) in Multiple Sclerosis (MS): 942. Official journal of the American College of Gastroenterology | ACG. 2011 Oct;106:S352.

59. Makkawi S, Camara-Lemarroy C, Metz L. Fecal microbiota transplantation associated with 10 years of stability in a patient with SPMS. Neurology - Neuroimmunology Neuroinflammation (Internet). 2018 Jul 1 (cited 2022 Mar 3);5(4). Available from: https://nn.neurology.org/content/5/4/e459

60. Borody T, Campbell J, Torres M, Nowak A, Leis S. Reversal of Idiopathic Thrombocytopenic Purpura (ITP) with Fecal Microbiota Transplantation (FMT): 941. Official journal of the American College of Gastroenterology | ACG. 2011 Oct;106:S352.

61. Zeng J, Peng L, Zheng W, Huang F, Zhang N, Wu D, et al. Fecal microbiota transplantation for rheumatoid arthritis: A case report. Clinical Case Reports. 2021;9(2):906–9.

62. Lawson Health Research Institute. Fecal Microbial Transplantation in Relapsing Multiple Sclerosis Patients (Internet). clinicaltrials.gov; 2019 Nov (cited 2022 Mar 1). Report No.: study/NCT03183869. Available from: https://clinicaltrials.gov/ct2/show/study/NCT03183869

63. Kragsnaes MS, Kjeldsen J, Horn HC, Munk HL, Pedersen JK, Just SA, et al. Safety and efficacy of faecal microbiota transplantation for active peripheral psoriatic arthritis: an exploratory randomised placebo-controlled trial. Annals of the Rheumatic Diseases. 2021 Sep 1;80(9):1158–67.

64. Borody T, Torres M, Campbell J, Hills L, Ketheeswaran S. Treatment of Severe Constipation Improves Parkinson's Disease (PD) Symptoms: 999. Official journal of the American College of Gastroenterology | ACG. 2009 Oct;104:S367.

65. Silva YP, Bernardi A, Frozza RL. The Role of Short-Chain Fatty Acids From Gut Microbiota in Gut-Brain Communication. Frontiers in Endocrinology (Internet). 2020 (cited 2022 Mar 8);11. Available from: https://www.frontiersin.org/article/10.3389/fendo.2020.00025

66. Sun MF, Zhu YL, Zhou ZL, Jia XB, Xu YD, Yang Q, et al. Neuroprotective effects of fecal microbiota transplantation on MPTP-induced Parkinson's disease mice: Gut microbiota, glial reaction and TLR4/TNF-α signaling pathway. Brain, Behavior, and Immunity. 2018 May 1;70:48–60.

67. Zhao Z, Ning J, Bao X Qi, Shang M, Ma J, Li G, et al. Fecal microbiota transplantation protects rotenone-induced Parkinson's disease mice via suppressing inflammation mediated by the lipopolysaccharide-TLR4 signaling pathway through the microbiota-gut-brain axis. Microbiome. 2021 Nov 17;9(1):226.

68. Harach T, Marungruang N, Duthilleul N, Cheatham V, Mc Coy KD, Frisoni G, et al. Reduction of Abeta amyloid pathology in APPPS1 transgenic mice in the absence of gut microbiota. Sci Rep. 2017 Feb 8;7(1):41802.

69. Sun J, Xu J, Ling Y, Wang F, Gong T, Yang C, et al. Fecal microbiota transplantation alleviated Alzheimer's disease-like pathogenesis in APP/PS1 transgenic mice. Transl Psychiatry. 2019 Aug 5;9(1):1–13.

70. Sun MF, Shen YQ. Dysbiosis of gut microbiota and microbial metabolites in Parkinson's Disease. Ageing Research Reviews. 2018 Aug 1;45:53–61.

71. Huang H, Xu H, Luo Q, He J, Li M, Chen H, et al. Fecal microbiota transplantation to treat Parkinson's disease with constipation. Medicine (Baltimore). 2019 Jun 28;98(26):e16163.

72. Xue LJ, Yang XZ, Tong Q, Shen P, Ma SJ, Wu SN, et al. Fecal microbiota transplantation therapy for Parkinson's disease. Medicine (Baltimore). 2020 Aug 28;99(35):e22035.

73. Segal A, Zlotnik Y, Moyal-Atias K, Abuhasira R, Ifergane G. Fecal microbiota transplant as a potential treatment for Parkinson's disease – A case series. Clinical Neurology and Neurosurgery. 2021 Aug 1;207:106791.

74. Kuai X Yi, Yao X Han, Xu L Juan, Zhou Y Qing, Zhang L Ping, Liu Y, et al. Evaluation of fecal microbiota transplantation in Parkinson's disease patients with constipation. Microbial Cell Factories. 2021 May 13;20(1):98.

75. Hazan S. Rapid improvement in Alzheimer's disease symptoms following fecal microbiota transplantation: a case report. J Int Med Res. 2020 Jun 1;48(6):0300060520925930.

76. Park SH, Lee JH, Shin J, Kim JS, Cha B, Lee S, et al. Cognitive function improvement after fecal microbiota transplantation in Alzheimer's dementia patient: a case report. Current Medical Research and Opinion. 2021 Oct 3;37(10):1739–44.

77. Kingston-Smith H, Clancy A, Holsinger D, Thomas J Borody. Treatment of Alzheimer's disease with combined antibiotics. In Hotel Grand Chancellor, Hobart, Tasmania: Australian Dementia Forum; 2019.

78. Sandler RH, Finegold SM, Bolte ER, Buchanan CP, Maxwell AP, Väisänen ML, et al. Short-term benefit from oral vancomycin treatment of regressive-onset autism. J Child Neurol. 2000 Jul;15(7):429–35.

79. Finegold SM, Molitoris D, Song Y, Liu C, Vaisanen ML, Bolte E, et al. Gastrointestinal microflora studies in late-onset autism. Clin Infect Dis. 2002 Sep 1;35(Suppl 1):S6–16.

80. Ahmed SA, Elhefnawy AM, Azouz HG, Roshdy YS, Ashry MH, Ibrahim AE, et al. Study of the gut Microbiome Profile in Children with Autism Spectrum Disorder: a Single Tertiary Hospital Experience. J Mol Neurosci. 2020 Jun 1;70(6):887–96.

81. Bermudez-Martin P, Becker JAJ, Caramello N, Fernandez SP, Costa-Campos R, Canaguier J, et al. The microbial metabolite p-Cresol induces autistic-like behaviors in mice by remodeling the gut microbiota. Microbiome. 2021 Jul 8;9(1):157.

82. Abuaish S, Al-Otaibi NM, Aabed K, Abujamel TS, Alzahrani SA, Alotaibi SM, et al. The Efficacy of Fecal Transplantation and *Bifidobacterium* Supplementation in Ameliorating Propionic Acid-Induced Behavioral and Biochemical Autistic Features in Juvenile Male Rats. J Mol Neurosci. 2022 Feb 1;72(2):372–81.

83. Nettleton JE, Klancic T, Schick A, Choo AC, Cheng N, Shearer J, et al. Prebiotic, Probiotic, and Synbiotic Consumption Alter Behavioral Variables and Intestinal Permeability and Microbiota in BTBR Mice. Microorganisms. 2021 Sep;9(9):1833.

84. Ramirez PL, Barnhill K, Gutierrez A, Schutte C, Hewitson L. Improvements in Behavioral Symptoms following Antibiotic Therapy in a 14-Year-Old Male with Autism. Case Reports in Psychiatry. 2013 Jun 19;2013:e239034.

85. Clancy AK, Gunaratne AW, Dolai S, Borody TJ. S1914 Antibiotics Followed by an Ultra Filtrate Fecal Microbiota Transplantation Improves Symptoms of Autism in an Adult Male. Official journal of the American College of Gastroenterology | ACG. 2021 Oct;116:S840.

86. Li N, Chen H, Cheng Y, Xu F, Ruan G, Ying S, et al. Fecal Microbiota Transplantation Relieves Gastrointestinal and Autism Symptoms by Improving the Gut Microbiota in an Open-Label Study. Front Cell Infect Microbiol. 2021 Oct 19;11:759435.

87. Kang DW, Adams JB, Coleman DM, Pollard EL, Maldonado J, McDonough-Means S, et al. Long-term benefit of Microbiota Transfer Therapy on autism symptoms and gut microbiota. Sci Rep. 2019 Apr 9;9(1):5821.

88. Lowy FD. Antimicrobial resistance: the example of *Staphylococcus aureus*. J Clin Invest. 2003 May 1;111(9):1265–73.

89. Gottfried J. History Repeating? Avoiding a Return to the Pre-Antibiotic Age (Internet). Harvard Law School Library; 2005 (cited 2022 Oct 4). Available from: https://dash.harvard.edu/bitstream/handle/1/8889467/Gottfried05.html

90. Levine DP. Vancomycin: A History. Clinical Infectious Diseases. 2006 Jan 1;42(Supplement_1):S5–12.

91. Wiley.com (Internet). (cited 2022 Oct 5). Miracle Cure: The Story of Penicillin and the Golden Age of Antibiotics | Wiley. Available from: https://www.wiley.com/en-sgMiracle+Cure%3A+The+Story+of+Penicillin+and+the+Golden+Age+of+Antibiotics-p-9780631164920

92. Biblio.com (Internet). (cited 2022 Oct 5). The Battle Against Bacteria: A Fresh Look by Peter Baldry - 1976. Available from: https://www.biblio.com/book/battle-against-bacteria-fresh-look-peter/d/1371186523

93. O'Callaghan A, van Sinderen D. Bifidobacteria and Their Role as Members of the Human Gut Microbiota. Front Microbiol. 2016 Jun 15;7:925.

94. Cheikhyoussef A, Pogori N, Chen W, Zhang H. Antimicrobial proteinaceous compounds obtained from bifidobacteria: From production to their application. International Journal of Food Microbiology. 2008 Jul;125(3):215–22.

95. Brüssow H. Problems with the concept of gut microbiota dysbiosis. Microbial Biotechnology. 2020;13(2):423–34.

96. Sokol H, Lay C, Seksik P, Tannock GW. Analysis of bacterial bowel communities of IBD patients: what has it revealed? Inflamm Bowel Dis. 2008 Jun;14(6):858–67.

97. Nguyen GC. Editorial: bugs and drugs: insights into the pathogenesis of inflammatory bowel disease. Am J Gastroenterol. 2011 Dec;106(12):2143–5.

98. Ng KM, Aranda-Díaz A, Tropini C, Frankel MR, Van Treuren W, O'Loughlin CT, et al. Recovery of the Gut Microbiota after Antibiotics Depends on Host Diet, Community Context, and Environmental Reservoirs. Cell Host & Microbe. 2019 Nov 13;26(5):650-665.e4.

99. Duncan K, Carey-Ewend K, Vaishnava S. Spatial analysis of gut microbiome reveals a distinct ecological niche associated with the mucus layer. Gut Microbes. 2021 Jan 1;13(1):1874815.

100. Normington C, Moura IB, Bryant JA, Ewin DJ, Clark EV, Kettle MJ, et al. Biofilms harbour *Clostridioides difficile*, serving as a reservoir for recurrent infection. npj Biofilms Microbiomes. 2021 Feb 5;7(1):1–10.

101. Chng KR, Ghosh TS, Tan YH, Nandi T, Lee IR, Ng AHQ, et al. Metagenome-wide association analysis identifies microbial determinants of post-antibiotic ecological recovery in the gut Nat Ecol Evol. 2020 Sep;4(9):1256–67.

102. Gibbons SM. Keystone taxa indispensable for microbiome recovery. Nat Microbiol. 2020 Sep;5(9):1067–8.

ACKNOWLEDGEMENTS

This book would not have been possible without the trillions of microbes that inhabit our bodies—our silent companions, guardians, and at times, instigators. Their roles in shaping human health continue to astonish, and it has been a privilege to bring their story to life.

To my team at the Centre for Digestive Diseases and Axent Medical, thank you for your tireless work, analytical rigor, and late-night brainstorms. Your dedication to advancing microbiome science is the engine behind every page of this book.

I would like to express my heartfelt gratitude to Dr Siba Dolai, whose dedication, precision, and passion for the microbiome made this work a reality. Dr Dolai was instrumental in organising the research materials, coordinating video interviews, and working closely with me to review and update the manuscript. His scientific insight and leadership throughout the writing process were invaluable.

A special thanks to Dr John Ng, who authored most of the initial draft. His ability to synthesize scientific complexity into readable narratives laid the foundation for this book. I also wish to acknowledge Jasmine Sandes for her editorial contribution—her attention to clarity and flow brought a polished cohesiveness to the early manuscript.

My deepest appreciation goes to Dr Will Davies, the principal editor of this book, who brought a transformative editorial touch to the work. Dr Davies restructured and refined the content with exceptional skill, turning a dense scientific narrative into a compelling and accessible story—one that welcomes not just scientists, but anyone curious about the microscopic world within.

And finally, my sincere thanks to our publisher, Mick Le Moignan of Bouley Bay Books for his substantial edit, foreword and contributions to the inclusions and layout, and to Trish Le Moignan for the graphics and cover artwork.

To the many patients, clinicians, and researchers who have walked this journey with me—thank you for your stories, your courage, and your questions. And to the microbes: thank you for teaching us that sometimes, healing starts at the bottom.

Prof Thomas Borody